# Anxiety: Panicking about Panic

## A powerful, self-help guide for those suffering from an Anxiety or Panic Disorder

Joshua Fletcher

Anxiety: Panicking about Panic. A powerful, self-help guide for those suffering from an Anxiety and Panic Disorder
Copyright © 2014 by Joshua Fletcher

## Dedication

I dedicate this book to Harry. Thank you for your inspiration during the happiest and darkest of times.

## Acknowledgements

I would like to acknowledge the input of many anxiety sufferers from around the world who have shared their stories and experiences through various blogs and forums. These experiences, whether positive or negative, have contributed towards my understanding of the condition and have helped me to write this book.

I would also like to thank Hannah for helping me to edit this book and supporting me through some difficult and challenging times. Your support has been invaluable and I'm lucky to share my life with you.

# Contents

## PART 4

# Introduction

Hello and thank you for purchasing this book. My name is Josh and for years I suffered with anxiety and unexplainable panic. In April 2012, after confidently stating that I was free from the clutches of excessive anxiety, I decided to write this self-help book for similar people who are struggling with anxiety, worry, panic attacks and the constant overwhelming feeling of fear and dread. This book is strongly tailored towards those who are suffering from a panic disorder or a debilitating anxiety condition.

If you struggle with anxiety and panic, or are perhaps suffering at this very moment, then fear not as this book has been purposely constructed to quickly put your mind at ease. I know that reading or focusing on anything can be difficult when feeling panicky or 'on edge', but stick with me on this one and I assure you that this book has the tools to help you alleviate your current fears. No matter how long you've been suffering for – weeks, months or even years – an anxiety and panic problem can be fixed.

Anxiety, panic and irrational thoughts are debilitating and scary, leading us into depressive states because we believe that we do not function properly as valued human beings with it seemingly ever present. However, just by opening this book, you have given clear evidence that you're striving to do something about this ongoing problem, which in itself is incredibly brave thing to do. It's also proof that you're not going 'insane' – a common symptom/assumption that many people seem to conclude when battling anxiety – because you've acknowledged something isn't right and by picking up this book you've made a rational, conscious choice to do something about it.

I've written this book as an 'easy to access', self-help guide for those whose lives have been severely affected by panic and the symptoms of anxiety. It has been written from a perspective that takes into regard my own battle with anxiety, as well as using knowledge that has been built up through observations and working with other sufferers.

This book begins with a comprehensive list of symptoms that relate to anxiety, although it primarily addresses anxiety's main symptoms which consist of unexplainable panic, panic attacks, derealisation, hypochondria, continuous fear and hypersensitivity. I believe that these are the root cause of all of the other physical problems that can arise with anxiety, such as heart palpitations, chest pains, headaches, insomnia, dizziness etc.

This book is then split into four main parts: the first part covers the basics of anxiety, panic and what's happening within our mind and bodies when we find ourselves panicking. It's probable you'll find that reading this part of the book imparts a strong form of relief, as it provides an essential tool needed for the recovery process – an understanding of what's actually going on.

Part two is a detailed list of the symptoms that can occur with anxiety. It is set out using a *'What?'* and *'Why?'* format to simplify and explain why such symptoms occur.

Part three offers further information and practical advice to keep anxiety and panic at bay and part four is a short 'emergency relief' section written for those who are experiencing a panic attack.

So let us begin. Give this book a chance and I'm sure it will help ten-fold to put your mind at ease.

*Worry never robs tomorrow of it's sorrow, it only saps today of it's joy –*
Leo Buscaglia

# The Symptoms of an Anxiety and Panic problem

## Psychological symptoms:

- **Excessive Worry**
- **Panic Attacks**
- **Derealisation** (feeling lucid and detached from surroundings)
- **Depersonalisation** (feeling detached from persona/personality)
- **Feeling apprehensive**
- **Hypochondria** (The fear that you're seriously ill)
- **The fear of a panic attack**
- **Body checking** (Looking for illness)
- **Repetitive & looping thoughts**
- **Feeling terrified**
- **Obsessive thoughts**
- **Inability to relax**
- **Difficulty completing tasks**
- **Feeling hopeless and depressed**
- **Overactive imagination**
- **Agoraphobia** (fear of going outside)

- Fear of other people's opinions
- Fear of embarrassment
- Fear that you're developing a psychological illness
- Self-analysing (checking the body for signs that something is wrong)
- Negative thoughts of isolation
- Deep level of focus about personal 'identity'
- Loss of appetite
- Big increase in appetite
- Loss of libido
- Loss of interest in work
- Loss of interest doing things that were once enjoyable
- Depressive thoughts
- Dwelling on thoughts
- Constantly trying to work out how to feel 'normal' again
- Constantly feeling tired
- Dampened sense of humor
- Inability to focus

# Physical symptoms:

- Heart palpitations (short bursts of a rapid heartbeat)
- Headaches – constant or recurring
- Light headedness
- Exhaustion
- Constant lethargy

- Irregular bowel movements
- **Chest pains** (ache)
- **Chest pains** (sharp stabbing)
- **Bloating**
- **Tickling/fluttering sensation in chest and esophagus**
- **Nausea**
- **Constant pacing**
- **Dizziness**
- **Perspiration** (sweating frequently)
- **Tinnitus** (ringing ears)
- **Stomach cramps**
- **Eye floaters** (particle-like objects that 'float' in front of vision)
- **Symptoms of Irritable Bowel Syndrome**
- **Rib pains**
- **Rib discomfort** (feeling pressure under ribs)
- **Stomach grumbling**
- **Dry mouth**
- **Feeling tired after eating**
- **Abdominal pains**
- **Shooting pains in back and abdomen**
- **Neck ache and pains**
- **Ache behind eyes**
- **Erectile dysfunction**
- **Jaw ache and tenderness**

# PART 1

## 1.1 Do I have an anxiety problem?

You're reading this book, albeit through probable desperation, because you've acknowledged the fact that something isn't quite right with your mind and body. Perhaps you don't feel like the way that you 'used to', and that your days are often dictated by odd feelings of apprehension and worry. It's also likely that you've often found yourself being struck with bouts of unexplainable panic, which can often trigger a chain of events where you may ultimately begin to panic about the state of panicking itself.

On top of anxious thoughts and panic attacks, maybe you're experiencing the feelings of constant worry, states of derealisation (detachment from self and surroundings), an inability to relax, strange bodily changes and depression. Believe it or not but these are all common symptoms of an unbelievably non-complex anxiety condition. Anxiety actually has an overabundance of symptoms, some of which you may have stumbled across at the start of this book. These symptoms, which range from the obvious to the obscure, are all linked with anxiety in some way.

I suggest that you take a look at the comprehensive list and see which of the symptoms can be applied to you and your current state. A lot of these symptoms crop up almost exclusively alongside an ongoing anxiety condition, and have direct links with suffering from an anxiety or panic disorder.

Anxiety comes with a lot of baggage and to the uneducated victim it can be a confusing and frightening condition. After my first run in with anxiety it didn't take long for me to desperately start foraging for an answer to explain how and why I felt the way I did – a decision which saw my anxiety worsen before it got better. I will explain in depth later on.

'Anxiety' is a word/topic that floats around society and dips in and out of conversation as frequently as talking about the weather. Take these for example: *"I'm anxious about my upcoming interview"*, *"My partner's absence is giving me anxiety"*, *"I can't wait until this is over so I can relax"*, *"This is nail-biting stuff!"* are all common examples of phrases that occur in conversation as a way to describe the way a person is feeling due to a fear of a possible outcome.

This type of anxiety doesn't seem to be questioned because throughout our lives we have concluded that this type of anxiety is normal. It is *normal* to fear an exam result, the dentist, an operation, public speaking, what the boss will say etc. However, when worrying thoughts and anxious behavior become a daily constant - for reasons beyond our comprehension - we start to acknowledge and admit to ourselves that something isn't quite right.

The classic and most common sign of an anxiety problem is when we find that our days are mostly being dictated by feelings of intense and unexplainable fear, and that we may begin to perceive everything around us as different and somewhat 'detached'. Further to this, panic may have crept into our lives, which can act as a focus point for our worries to be directed towards. This fear can easily lead us to questioning things such as our health, our perception of reality and believing in the most unlikely of worst case scenarios.

Below are some of the common assumptions that the standard anxiety victim can often relate to:

# Anxiety Assumptions

- I feel terrified for no logical reason.

- I haven't felt normal for a long time, something must be wrong.

- Why am I scared to do 'normal' things?

- A psychological condition must be the cause for this change.

- I must have a serious health problem. I.e. Heart failure, Cancer.

- My brain/mind does not work like those around me.

- I don't think this is ever going to go away. I can't handle it.

- No one else fully understands what I'm going through.

- Why do I feel like I'm about to die?

Furthermore, it is important that we look at some of the most common *physical* symptoms that signal an anxiety problem. The symptoms section at the start of this book supplies a comprehensive list of symptoms that have all been linked to anxiety; below are some I have found to be the most common:

### The Most Common Physical Symptoms

- **Heart** - Palpitations, chest flutters, 'skipping a beat', heart pounding, hyperawareness of heart beat.

- **Abdominal Pains** - Chest pains and tightness, stomach pains and cramping.

- **Derealisation** - sense of unreality, an illusory detachment from surroundings, shut down of peripheral vision, difficulty focusing.

- **Head** - Constant and prolonged headaches, light headedness, dizziness, vertigo, tinnitus, sensitivity to light, eye floaters

- **Energy** - Tiredness, lethargy, 'heavy head', exhaustion

- **Pain** - Unfamiliar aches and pains, cramps, rib pain, muscle tension pain, dental pain

- **I.B.S** - Indigestion, constipation, acid reflux, trapped wind, diarrhoea, gut and intestinal pains.

If you feel that you can relate to any of the listed anxiety assumptions, and to several of the symptoms listed here and at the start of this book, then it would be a pretty safe bet to assume that you have an anxiety problem.

Fear not as an anxiety problem isn't at all dangerous; it cannot permanently harm you, and is something that's easily fixable when fully understood. What has happened - putting it in the most basic of terms - is that your body has arrived at a state of chemical imbalance as a result of trying to deal with high amounts stress and operating using a poor mental routine. In other words, unexplainable anxiety is your body's way of telling you that it has simply had enough and something has to change.

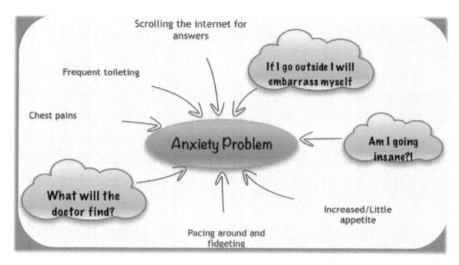

Let's take a look at these anxiety maps that represent some common situations relating to anxiety. I highly recommend making your own as it's a healthy, cathartic way of putting worries on paper. It also helps to clarify and organize problems into one accessible picture.

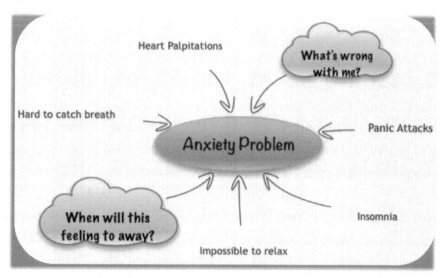

As you can see the 'Anxiety Problem' takes centre stage in the diagram and links all sorts of anxiety symptoms together. You'll find that a large array of symptoms can surround the core issue of the anxiety problem - particularly those symptoms that feel somewhat 'new' to the person who is experiencing it.

I suggest that at some point, when you feel that you can, you should write down everything that worries you and place all of these worries into an anxiety map like the ones featured here. I honestly can't emphasize enough how such a simple task ends up becoming an enlightening and powerful form of relief. Why not trial pointing your physical and psychological ailments to anxiety? Hopefully you'd have discovered a strong link here.

I, like many others, fell into the trap of assuming the worse about my predicament. *'Something must be wrong with me,'* I often thought, usually spending the majority of my day analysing why I felt the way I did and panicking when the feelings didn't go away. All that I was experiencing was **anxiety** - an unbelievably non-complex condition (despite its many horrible symptoms) that is harmless and easily overcome.

It's important to know that a common feeling that accompanies an anxiety disorder is the feeling of being 'stuck' or trapped in a constant loop of worrying thoughts and panic. When this happens we may start to become anxious for reasons beyond our normal ability to rationalise. We start to dwell on why we feel panicky and are inevitably sucked into the dark world of high anxiety and the increasing likelihood of panic attacks.

Ultimately, we can start to become anxious *because* we are feeling anxious. We can begin to question the very reason why we feel the way we do, and if you're like the 'old' me you probably spend every day doing just this. Every day!

It doesn't take a genius to work out that anxious thoughts and questioning the way you feel can easily become an unwanted, obsessive hobby. You're probably doing it now, or it's queued in your thought pattern somewhere.

This obsessive behavior can easily spill over and dictate our actions too. Perhaps you've spent days on end perilously researching your symptoms on search engines, only to find that you've been frightened by what you've discovered despite the obvious improbability. When we are anxious, we become vulnerable and are easily drawn to the worst case scenario in a given situation. Search engines often have the habit of churning out fatalistic diagnoses and stories of isolated misfortune. Unfortunately, when we are vulnerable, we are drawn to this information which provides only negativity to feed our obsessions.

I know it's extremely hard to put scary and repetitive thoughts aside but for now at least, just let it go. Nothing bad will happen to you. 'Bad' is a subjective term, but I deem 'bad' in relation to the topic of anxiety as the feeling like you're about to die, or something awful is about to happen. Always remember that feeling anxious cannot do this to you.

A common problem with anxiety is that it feels like it's tailored to the individual. The longer the strange feelings and symptoms continue, the more likely we assume something is wrong upstairs. By 'upstairs' I mean our constantly ticking, never resting brains. One day we're feeling fine, then the next day we feel completely different and the world around us also feels and appears different. We fall prey to our feelings and emotions and our reality becomes a superficial projection of what's actually going on.

I, like many others I have helped and likewise have helped me, found it such a relief when being able to identify and relate to the symptoms which can occur with anxiety. Some of these symptoms present as very strange and may have you questioning why and if they relate to anxiety at all. The simple answer is that when we are in an anxious state, our body operates on a different level, and over time this different 'mode' of operation takes its toll on the body and mind.

This is all to do with adrenaline and other bodily chemicals which will be explained in depth later on. Rest assured, these symptoms are common, and to further ease your worries I have set out a chapter later in this book dedicated to explaining each symptom to you.

# The Anxiety Umbrella

The first step any anxiety sufferer should take is to simplify their chaotic world of worries. It unfortunately took me three years to work this out - something that will take you the duration of an afternoon - but rest assured it helped me tenfold to tame my constant worry. It's the first step that should be taken when beginning to take control of anxiety.

When anxiety is high and blinding confusion has set in, you'll know that it can be extremely difficult to prioritise, organise and focus on your 'problems' in any logical order or with any rational sense. We have so many different worries, which amount on top of our underlying worry of 'not feeling right', that we simply just don't know where to start. Have you tried waiting for the feelings to go away? You'll know it simply does not work like that.

Take a look at the examples of types of worries on the next page:

| Daily Life Worries | Social Worries | Worries from Perspective |
|---|---|---|
| • Work / Job<br>• Bills<br>• Finance<br>• Education<br>• Domestic Jobs<br>• Appointments<br>• Security<br>• Deadlines<br>• Examinations<br>• Unenjoyable tasks.<br>• Chores | • Relationships<br>• Friendships<br>• Family<br>• Parenthood<br>• Social Circles<br>• Confidence<br>• Loss of Sense of Humour<br>• Expectations<br>• Judgement | • Religious perspective<br>• Philosophical outlook<br>• Life purpose/meaning<br>• Self Worth<br>• Over analysing situations<br>• Misanthropy<br>• 'The outside world is a scary place'<br>• 'Nobody understands what I 'm going through' |

## Hypochondria (Health Worries)

- 'Am I going insane?'
- Self analysing
- Body checking for problems.
- Fear of having a panic attack
- Convinced of having a heart problem, cancer, schizophrenia, etc.
- Questioning aches, pains, twinges and assuming the worst.

Now let's scatter a few examples around in a similar fashion to the anxiety maps. I once again suggest that you take this opportunity to use your own experiences whilst utilizing these examples as a guideline.

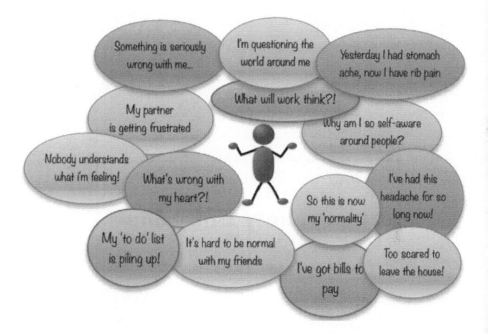

Can you see how hard it must be to prioritise a single worry to deal with? Where do we even start?

Of course it's normal to have every day worries such as work and social issues, however these worries can soon multiply and increase in intensity when anxiety is present. Anxiety can soon act as a barrier to resolving every day issues, which results in worries building up very quickly. Worries and stress become harder to resolve causing an accumulation effect similar to that of the common snowball analogy.

The key here, which forms as one of the core foundations of this book, is to group everything as one problem - the problem being the simplified term 'anxiety'. Take everything that you've ever assumed and worried about with regards to how you feel and throw it under a metaphorical umbrella. Label it 'anxiety' and voila – your problems are simplified to one manageable problem.

*'What do I do with this umbrella?'* you may ask. Well I've written this book to tell you. If I'd have known all that time ago that all I was experiencing was symptoms of anxiety I'd have saved myself a hell of a lot of time and energy. Five years worth of time to be more precise.

Let us take a look at this poorly drawn anxiety umbrella for sake of clarity (drawing is not my forte):

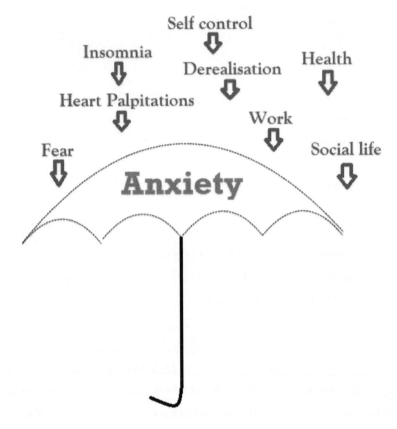

As you can see, the umbrella symbolizes anxiety as a whole and the 'rain drops' symbolize some of the components or symptoms that form an anxiety condition. Instead of trying to deal with every issue or symptom separately, I challenge you to try and allow all of your worries to be associated with anxiety. This not only simplifies the problem, it allows room for reflection and a point of 'blame' if life simply becomes too much.

# I'm handing out labels and pills. Who wants some?

In the introduction I referred to the term 'anxiety' from a more generalised perspective, when in fact it acts as more of a forename for a plethora of conditions which fall under several different subcategories. Here is a list of conditions which will most likely seem familiar to you or you may cross paths with at some point:

- Generalised Anxiety Disorder (GAD)
- Panic Disorder
- Health Anxiety Disorder
- Obsessive Compulsive Disorder
- Anxiety and Depressive Disorder
- Agoraphobia
- Social Anxiety
- Retroactive Jealousy

Of course there are other strands of anxiety that fall under different categories, but the list above consists of the names that tend to float around the most. Furthermore, I can openly admit that each of the labels listed could, at one time, be associated as a condition that I have personally experienced and been through.

We sometimes put labels on ourselves to provide some false sense of understanding about what we're confused about. It acts as a comfort blanket and simplifies complex issues that we're unsure of or uneducated in. I'm not boldly stating that you have been misdiagnosed, and that I am contradicting the views of a trained medical professional, but what's remarkable about what I have found in my research is the importance sufferers place on possessing a medical label to make sense of what appears to be a complex problem.

A large proportion of the anxiety sufferers I have worked with use these labels to make sense of something they fear, therefore taking the 'edge' of an issue that they find incredibly scary. Look at these for example:

- ❖ **"I can't go outside because I suffer from *Agoraphobia*"**
- ❖ **"I have a *Panic Disorder* so I can't attend the event"**
- ❖ **"When this *Depression* leaves I can return to my normal life"**
- ❖ **"I wish I could do all these things but I have an *Anxiety Disorder*"**
- ❖ **"Don't blame me it's my *O.C.D*"**

So... If you can relate to anything this book has mentioned so far then I throw down the gauntlet to you - I dare you to lose any labels you've attributed to yourself and simply blame everything on anxiety. The advantage of openly acknowledging you have an anxiety 'condition' is that conditions can be changed. It is merely temporary.

You could argue that acknowledging you have an anxiety condition is much like giving yourself a new label. However, I'm asking you to acknowledge anxiety as a changeable condition – one that can be immediately challenged and laid to rest.

The first thing I had to do to tackle my anxiety was to lose the labels I held above my head and structured my life around. I *knew* I was depressed, I *knew* I was scared to leave the house and I *knew* things were a lot different from before.

What I realised is that it wasn't the medical condition crippling me, but the constant and overwhelming *fear* that overcame me on a daily basis. After much deep thought I decided that if a medical condition was to dictate my life it could do so, but I was in no way going to let my life be dictated by a negative emotion. Fear was not going to dictate my life. Fear is an emotion, not a medical condition.

An anxiety problem can be fixed with understanding and good practice; before long you'll be living a life free from the clutches of gripping fear and worry. I sit here today laughing at the years I spent trapped in this loop of high anxiety and panic, but at the same time I know that I could have saved years of my life if I had been educated earlier.

This is where I feel a lot of the problems lie in terms of anxiety becoming out of hand for a lot of people. Focusing on the health profession's role within the world of anxiety; it is in my and many others' opinion that certain sectors of the health profession (not excluding the excellent work done by many in the profession and within mental health) approach anxiety with too much haste and misunderstanding. Many people feel that the common referral processes, combined with an overloaded demand for access to services, can often lead to misdiagnosis, mistreatment and a lack of time assessing the individual and their needs.

Perhaps like me you've sampled the many medicinal approaches to treating anxiety such as anti-depressants, pseudo drugs, herbal remedies and 'miracle cures'. Once again I'm not in a position to state the positive benefits of such medicines, but what I can share with you is that I - and many others I have helped - found that these drugs did not help at all in terms of easing the symptoms of anxiety and the underlying fear that accompanies it.

Drugs such as anti-depressants are undoubtedly designed to change how we feel. When we are anxious we are vulnerable to states of hypersensitivity - meaning that we're alert to any change in ourselves and our environment. This is why it's commonly found that anti-depressants don't allow anxiety victims to get to the core of the problem. We often spend a lot of time scanning ourselves to see if we're 'ok', but with drugs altering our current state of mind they can often end up causing the opposite of the intended outcome. We panic and over-think about everything that seems different within or around us. Ultimately, it heightens our sense of *losing control*.

I trust my general practitioner, and my CBT nurse, but overall I think the medical profession lacks the knowledge about the topic of anxiety as a whole and are too quick to throw pills at it alongside grouping it with depression. Anxiety is not depression. Anxiety can only lead to depression over time, or when someone has accepted that their future lies in the hands of solely feeling a certain way.

This is the reason behind writing this book. The answer to conquering your anxiety is pretty simple but has overwhelming results. All I ask of you is to ask yourself *'Do I have all of these separate problems?'*, or is it simply the question *'Do I have an anxiety problem?'*

# 1.2 Why am I panicking and where did this come from?

Constant overwhelming anxiety, quite unsurprisingly, is caused by the sufferer getting into a habit of too much worry. Over time excessive and continual worry creates a chemical imbalance within our bodies causing constant, unmeasured amounts of adrenaline and other chemicals to be released into our systems. These chemicals, in any measure, can and *will* cause noticeable changes in us both physically and mentally - particularly when adrenaline is released in large amounts on a frequent basis.

It's important to explain that quite often our biggest worry during these times is the constant awareness of feeling different from our usual selves and in a lot of cases feeling a detachment from our surroundings. This is called entering states of *depersonalization* and *derealisation*. These symptoms can be extremely discomforting and can often leave us feeling frightened. We can find ourselves rapidly foraging for an answer to the newly found problem - striving for order and an explanation for a feeling that we currently feel clueless about.

Like I mentioned before, the main culprit for these feelings is the wonderful chemical **adrenaline** - with the aid of other released bodily chemicals such as cortisol. These chemicals are primarily responsible for leading us into episodes of extreme panic, hypersensitivity, lucid derealisation and triggering concern about other physical symptoms. Adrenaline isn't a chemical to be feared however, it just needs to be understood.

Further to adrenaline affecting our bodies, when anxiety and panic strike frequently and continuously over time, it begins to over-stimulate our nervous systems. An over-stimulated nervous system sets us on high alert mode and it's more than common to feel hyperaware, hypersensitive and overly conscious of 'dangers' in our surroundings and even within our bodies. It's easy to become overly *aware* of our anxiety, our panic and how different we currently feel from our usual selves.

I realise that up to now there's a lot to take in, so let's break it down.

## Breaking it down:

❖ Poor thought patterns and a bad behavioral routine cause the body to release excessive amounts of adrenaline.

❖ Adrenaline causes various changes within our bodies and eventually causes a chemical imbalance.

❖ Over time a constant flow of adrenaline causes us to become hypersensitive and hyperaware of ourselves and our surroundings (Fight or Flight response).

❖ Adrenaline and hypersensitivity can cause us to experience episodes of depersonalisation and derealisation.

❖ Over time our nervous systems become over- stimulated making us further prone to anxiety and panic. We begin to panic about why we feel the way we do.

❖ We begin to panic about the other symptoms anxiety can cause (refer to symptoms list).

❖ We're stuck in a loop of worrying and panicking about our well-being and attaching our own reasoning to why we feel the way we do.

It may sound unmeasured, but all you need to know is that you have an **anxiety problem**. Or to put it in other words, you're failing to understand and accept what adrenaline is doing to your body. I'd suspect that almost all of your problems revolve around how you and your body react to dumps of adrenaline and how you re-enact negative thought and behaviour habits.

---

# Fight-or-Flight

A physiological reaction in response to stress, characterized by an increase in heart rate and blood pressure, elevation of glucose levels in the blood, and redistribution of blood from the digestive tract to the muscles. These changes are caused by activation of the sympathetic nervous system by epinephrine (adrenaline), which prepares the body to challenge or flee from a perceived threat.

-The American Heritage® Science Dictionary

---

Of course everyone experiences doses of adrenaline on a frequent basis. It is a normal bodily chemical that helps us function as human beings by triggering our 'fight or flight' response. However, when it becomes excessive - particularly when caused by stress, negative thoughts and behaviours - it can easily turn into a daily anxiety or panic problem. Instead of our days being 'normal' they can turn into prolonged battles against our own mind and body which is nothing short of exhausting.

It is of absolute importance to understand and accept that an anxiety problem and frequent panic attacks don't just occur overnight; it is the result of something that has built up over time. This could have started by worrying about personal and subjective issues, or triggered by a life event causing a traumatic effect on the body.

When these worries aren't dealt with or solved, they then unknowingly accumulate on top of one another causing the sufferer to reach their peak in terms of being in an anxious state. The sufferer (you) is stuck in a constant fluctuation between high anxiety and panic.

These worries then often evolve into *new* worries that revolve around well-being and the concept of suffering from a mental health condition, i.e. 'going insane'. Free-flowing adrenaline is being released in copious amounts - causing all sorts of changes both physically and mentally - and we're left in a bit of a mess. The next section goes into this in more detail.

But wait a second. A pretty grounded person would be intelligent enough to work out these feelings and emotions themselves, so why not do just that?

No, this would be a colossal error.

It's a common trap for many people when acknowledging something is wrong to then attempt to use seemingly harmless logic to try to 'solve' the anxiety problem. Another common trap is to simply wait for the feelings to go away.

Except that 'working it out' is just another worry added onto a giant smorgasbord of worries that we previously had. Panic then sets in because we have waited more than enough time for these feelings to disappear, but alas they linger and appear to become stronger than ever!

Then, to make things even more complicated, the physical symptoms that come hand in hand with worry start to appear. The headaches, stomach cramps, reality distortion, racing heart beats, shortness of breath, dizziness and sweating to name a mere few. What an even greater mess!

To put it simply, our anxiety is caused by a simple imbalance in the body caused by continuous stress or trauma. Adrenaline and other chemicals are released in disproportionate amounts causing us to feel strange and hypersensitive to aches, pains,other bodily changes and what's happening in our environment. Our nervous systems become over-stimulated, which further puts us on high alert and sensitive to changes in ourselves and our environment. However, as many of us are unaware of this, we are stuck worrying and questioning the way we feel and why we feel so scared. We become victims to our own hypersensitivity.

# The Loop of Peaking Anxiety

It is extremely important to understand that you don't just wake up with full blown anxiety. It is a condition that reveals its true colours over time and is often only consciously identifiable at it's **peak**. This means that the working cogs of your anxiety condition were put into motion at some point in the past and it is only now that you are aware that something is wrong because your anxiety is *peaking*.

This would explain why anxiety and panic attacks crop up from seemingly nowhere(my first panic attack struck when I was making a cup of tea at work). The peak of anxiety is often represented by sudden waves of anxiety, panic and an onslaught of the symptoms aforementioned at the start of this book. These symptoms can be ever present, they can also 'come and go', or they can be completely new to the sufferer as a result of a stressful week.

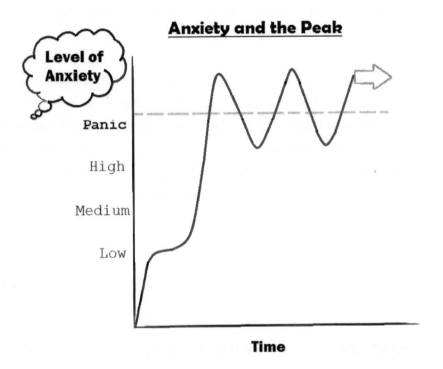

The overall result is a *loop* of anxious thoughts and relentless worry - something which I have labeled **The Loop of Peaking Anxiety**. I will use this diagram to provide more clarity:

Anything below the *Medium* level you would class as 'normal' anxiety - the worries that warrant an anxious response to issues found on a day to day basis. Note that even a high level of anxiety is normal, but when our anxiety exceeds this we are at risk of being struck with **panic**.

Unfortunately, it is common for many anxiety victims to be stuck fluctuating between high anxiety and panic, with the result being a traumatic 'loop' effect. Suddenly the normal day-to-day worries are not at the forefront of priorities anymore, with them being replaced by worries about our well-being and this newly formed anxious state.

Consider the following analogy:

Imagine your anxiety being channeled through an electrical plug. The electrical plug has a fuse which represents your body's ***coping mechanisms***. The more stress and worrying thoughts that you pile on yourself, then the stronger the power the plug's fuse has to deal with.

The stress and worry slowly builds up until your body simply can't take anymore. The fuse blows, the circuit shuts down and you're left in a confused mess trying to work out what exactly just happened. You can't operate like you used to anymore because there is nothing to control all of this surging 'power'.

The body's coping mechanisms - which consist of positive rationalization, your body's ability to maintain a chemical balance and the familiar feeling of accepting what you're used to – have completely gone, thus unveiling a bizarre world of terror and confusion. You are left to work out an answer to an unsolvable puzzle. You start to question why you feel the way you do, *why* it happened, finding your own irrational solutions etc. You can become stuck within the infamous loop! Fear not as this is easily fixed with the power of understanding.

To the unaware sufferer it can be very difficult to 'return' or settle down to normality again. It's not uncommon that people have lived with anxiety for years, stuck in the same looping habit of questioning why they feel the way they do, or just waiting for the feelings and thoughts to disappear.

Many victims, including myself at one time, make it depressing routine to constantly self analyse – firstly checking how we feel, then scanning our bodies for signs that there is something wrong. We do this because we're stuck in the *loop of peaking anxiety*.

We often resign ourselves to thinking we have an incurable, psychological condition because frankly we often conclude that nothing seems to be working. What we don't fully realise is that we're thinking out of *fear* and consciously looking for reasons to provide fabrication and meaning for this fear. One of the worst mistakes I made was to wake up and immediately think *"Do I feel better today?!"* Funnily enough I didn't.

Being stuck in a loop at the peak of your anxiety is debilitating, depressing and awfully scary. However, use the knowledge of why you feel this way to provide a small, comforting degree of inner content. You are not going insane and in fact what you're experiencing is alarmingly common. What's also assuring is that what your body is doing is only natural, so no matter how long you've had this condition I can assure you nothing 'bad' will happen as a result of it. You could be anxious for the next one hundred years and your death would not be directly anxiety related.

No matter how many times you lose your breath, feel your heart pounding, lose your balance, feel lightheaded or focus on an abnormality; remember that the anxiety will not kill you. Anxiety is harmless and merely tricks you into thinking the world is crumbling around you and that you're dying a depressing, isolated death.

Part 1.3 explains what's exactly happening to you and your body during episodes of high anxiety and panic. With the power of understanding you will realise that what is happening does not warrant the fear that accompanies it.

# Why does an anxiety problem start?

There are two simple reasons why anxiety starts and later becomes horribly excessive:

The first cause is a basic one and that's human habit. When we get into a habit of worrying and constantly troubling ourselves with undesirable thoughts, this eventually takes its toll on the body. Have you ever been labeled a 'worrier'? Or know somebody in your life who you would deem to be a worrier?

Cognitive Behavioural Therapy tells us that obsessive worrying about certain thoughts is just the inability to detach from or let go of a thought. If you cannot let go or lessen the importance of a thought, then the worry that accompanies it simply just sticks around striving for attention and piling up with other worries.

We get into a habit of worrying until the body becomes disturbed, causing all of this anxiety and its army of symptoms to occur. It took a very long time for me to acknowledge and admit to myself that I was a worrier. It required me to study my thought patterns for a long time.

The second cause is trauma. Trauma starts the anxiety problems in a similar fashion to the first cause, except it skips the build up and gives your body a raging fireball to deal with. Referring back to the analogy before, trauma basically tries pushing the equivalent of the national grid through the 'plug socket' causing an immediate blowout.

Trauma is usually started by an unexpected incident in life where the body is put into shock. I.e, the death of a loved one, personal injury or illness, exposure to a fear, loss of job, divorce, adultery, and so on. Your coping mechanisms are wiped out and become non-existent. You perceive life differently compared to before the trauma, and unsurprisingly your body has a major chemical imbalance. You feel different and of course you now want to know why.

It's an extremely important part of your recovery to acknowledge exactly where the anxiety has come from and why it is happening to you. It takes a lot of bravery to admit to yourself that perhaps you were doing something self inflicting - particularly if you're a pretty self-assured person who thinks you have a large degree of self-control in your life.

I unfortunately developed my anxiety as a young man with a pretty large ego. What I failed to acknowledge is that my thought patterns were very negative and damaging in terms of affecting my mental health. I developed anxiety as a result of a poor mental routine and then eventually having to deal with a shocking life event. I will explain more about my story later on in this book.

# 1.3 Anxiety is Adrenaline and a Sensitive Nervous System

I think the most influential factor in my recovery was forming an understanding of what was actually happening during the episodes of high anxiety and panic. Of course I was aware of the more obvious related symptoms such as the racing thoughts, a fast heart rate, difficulty maintaining steady breathing, light headedness and the odd aches and pains. But the real panic came from wondering where these symptoms actually came from and *why* they were happening to me.

Unfortunately, I made the ultimate mistake by falling into one of anxiety's most formidable traps. I began to *fear* anxiety. I began to fear feeling panicky and feeling different - something which firmly fixes you within the clutches of anxiety.

In section 1.2, I explained about how anxiety builds up, and when we let it build up enough we can easily become caught in the *loop of peaking anxiety.* We begin to dwell on frightening thoughts, which in turn adds to our overall anxious state. When we feel anxious our body reacts to these anxious and frightening thoughts by releasing chemicals such as adrenaline and cortisol.

Adrenaline is a funny little chemical. It is great in times of danger and acts as a great defence mechanism for the body by triggering our 'fight or flight' response. However, when we are stuck in a habit of dwelling on frightening thoughts in a situation where 'fight or flight' isn't needed then adrenaline seems to become our adversary.

Our brain and adrenal gland start to work together by releasing plenteous amounts of adrenaline at times where we don't *need* it - thus causing our bodies to react to the adrenaline, causing all of these strange symptoms to appear and temporarily alter our perception of reality. It is the *thoughts* that keep triggering the adrenal gland to release these chemicals. It is the negative thoughts - not the will for the feeling to stop - that keep the adrenaline pumping.

Think about it. Can you recall how you felt the last time you dealt with a large dose of adrenaline? Try and recall how much you were stuck in your own head the minutes before a job interview, a risky operation or even something leisurely like a first date. Adrenaline is pumping through your system and all you seem to focus on is the situation that is imminent and directly in front of you. It's exactly the same when we are stuck with an anxiety problem.

Adrenaline and other bodily chemicals swim around our veins - affecting everything that we're used to during a 'normal' day - and we're left worrying and questioning why we feel so different and *why* we are constantly worrying. There appears to be no plausible danger in front of us, yet our body prepares us for one by constantly triggering the 'fight or flight' response. This inevitably lead me to become stuck in the 'Loop of Peaking Anxiety'. Never underestimate the power of thoughts and how they affect the body over time.

Constantly worrying about why I felt the way I did just led to my body constantly releasing adrenaline into the bloodstream. Over time the worry inevitably lead to the intense presence of stress both mentally and physically. This caused yet more worry because I then started to focus on the physical changes my body was going through.

Adrenaline causes all sorts of changes within the body, and over time it's usually responsible for all sorts of strange and wonderful things that can occur. It is extremely important to know that, in relation to anxiety, adrenaline can be found to be primarily responsible for:

## Continuous Adrenaline can cause:

❖ Increase in heart rate / palpitations / pounding chest ("Fight or Flight")

❖ Sudden and continuous sense of derealisation / detachment from surroundings

❖ Racing, looping thoughts ("Fight or Flight")

❖ Difficulty maintaining steady breathing / shortness of breath ("Fight or Flight")

❖ Dizziness / Light headedness / vision distortion

❖ Excessive sweating / Hot flushes

❖ Muscle Tension ("Fight or Flight")

❖ Hypersensitivity

❖ Panic Attacks

I recall dwelling on constant headaches, abdominal pains, lack of sleep and why my surroundings felt detached from me. Furthermore, I used to focus obsessively on an array of symptoms found in the **symptom list** at the start of the book. Everything felt different from what it used to be like and I needed to know why. The difficulty was that I didn't accept that these feelings would only be temporary if I allowed the adrenaline and cortisol to run it's course and let my body restore a chemical balance.

The solution that we strive for is so simple, but we all can fall victim to our racing thoughts and pay too much attention to them. If we just allow adrenaline to run its course, then the feeling of normality will eventually return. 'Normality' returns faster and faster the more we get used to paying our negative thoughts and feelings zero attention.

# Panic Attacks

When anxiety is at its highest - where worrying thoughts, stress, tiredness and a damaging routine have taken their toll - we experience something called a panic attack. A panic attack can also occur when exposed to shock, sudden trauma or being exposed to something that scares us.

A lot of people use the term as a means of exaggeration when in conversation. For example, *'Wow you scared me! You almost gave me a panic attack!'* would undoubtedly be something that you've heard in your lifetime. An actual panic attack however feels nothing short of terrifying to the person who is experiencing it.

A panic attack is when an intense feeling of fear, dread, loss of control and entrapment overwhelms a person. There is usually no identifiable trigger and they seem to strike from seemingly nowhere (you have learned that this is untrue). Accompanying these feelings are thoughts of an imminent disaster, impending doom and even the fear of sudden death. The number of anxiety victims I have spoken to who have ended up in the emergency room with no explainable symptoms borders on the absurd!

A panic attack leads you down roads of irrational thinking, where even the most intelligent of people are forced to feel and believe in the most unlikely of outcomes. I used to whirl up in a panic over a chest flutter, head ache, differences in breathing, stomach cramps, detachment from surroundings, I.e. I will explain more in the next section entitled *Rationality and Worst Case Scenarios*.

Along with these feelings are other physical symptoms that occur when panic has struck. A panic attack causes our muscles to tense up, our peripheral vision to shut down (tunnel vision) and alters the way we breath - tricking us into thinking we're not getting enough oxygen. It also causes light headedness, dizziness and sometimes nausea. Below are the main symptoms and feelings that occur during a panic attack:

# Panic Attacks

- Sudden and intense fright.
- A sense of derealisation / detachment from surroundings
- Chest pains
- Pounding or thumping chest
- Fast heart rate
- Difficulty maintaining a steady pace of breathing
- An overwhelming urge to 'escape' or run away.
- Irrational thinking. I.e. *Am I going to die? Is this a heart attack? I must have a serious condition like cancer.*
- Chest fluttering / heart palpitations
- Racing thoughts and confusion
- The urge to do anything but be stationary. I.e. pace the room or squeeze an object.

- Tunnel Vision
- The need to 'escape'

A panic attack can occur when the body releases a large amount of unexpected adrenaline into the bloodstream. I mentioned before that adrenaline can cause all sorts of changes both physically and mentally, so if we're unprepared or 'caught off guard' by a newly released dump of adrenaline, then it could be expected of us to panic about this sudden change.

The panic comes from the **confusion** about what is happening and this works in tandem with a belief that you cannot cope. Adrenaline actually causes our minds to race and be filled with all sorts of thoughts and conclusions as to *why* we're panicking and *why* we're feeling strange.

This would explain why so many people are convinced that they're having a heart attack, or that they're going insane, or that they have an incurable condition, and so on. It is the adrenaline that affects our rationality during these periods of panic, thus causing them to turn into prolonged *panic attacks.*

These panic attacks don't last forever because the adrenal gland finally becomes exhausted and cannot release any further adrenaline. The reader should take comfort in the fact that a panic attack cannot last forever because of this and the feeling of normality will return - at least until the adrenal gland has recharged and we may unknowingly fall back into the same repetitive thought habit.

Let's take a look at the *Anxiety and the Peak* diagram from 1.1 and explore how panic attacks tie in with the loop of peaking anxiety:

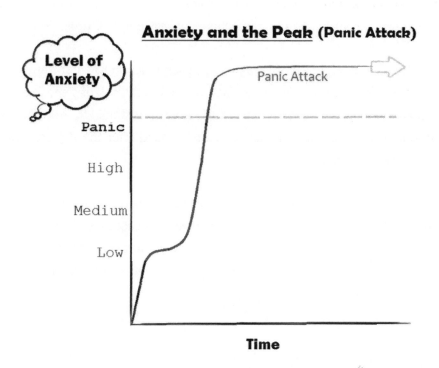

## Anxiety and the Peak (Panic Attack)

Instead of our anxiety and panic 'looping', a panic attack occurs when we're struck with a feeling of constant fear. To the person who experiences it the feeling can often feel like the fear is escalating or 'getting worse'. This is purely psychosomatic because a panic attack occurs at the peak of an adrenal outpour. In other words, and on a comforting note, once you're having a panic attack it can't get any 'worse' than when the attack initially strikes.

I, like many others, suffered my first panic attack in a situation where it appeared to creep up from seemingly nowhere. I was on my break at work, pouring myself a cup of tea, when I was suddenly struck and overwhelmed by a feeling of detachment from my surroundings. My breathing started to alter and I immediately felt worried as this feeling seemed so different to me. I inevitably started to panic; then I started to panic because I didn't know why I was panicking. I wanted normality to come straight back to me because I didn't feel in control of a situation where I usually am in control.

Simply put, a panic attack is just a chosen reaction to an unwanted dose of adrenaline. Stress, anxiety, fatigue, poor diet and lack of sleep lead to an imbalance within the body and our nervous systems to become over-stimulated. This causes adrenaline to be released after the slightest, almost unnoticeable trigger.

Use this knowledge and I assure you the next panic attack will not be half as bad. Since I learned this, the panic attacks became less and less intense and the duration decreased over a relatively short amount of time. I will provide further information and advice on dealing with panic attacks in the next part of this book.

# Rationality and Worst Case Scenarios

One of the most profound stumbling blocks that occur when trying to tackle anxiety is falling prey to our emotions and states of irrationality. When high states of panic and anxiety arise, a common thing we do as human beings is to try to work out what exactly is happening in order to make sense of a situation that can appear very confusing.

It is extremely important to acknowledge and realise that when anxiety is present, our normal sense of rationality can be massively distorted. Our thinking can become predominantly irrational due to the adrenaline that's flowing through our veins and implementing change in our bodies. We can become frightened at the possibility of something horrendous happening in any given situation. Trying to think rationally in 'fight or flight' mode is extremely tricky.

Take these scenarios for example: you're at home alone at night and you hear a loud bang, the first thing that commonly comes to mind is thinking is there an intruder in the house? Other examples include the scenario of your child not coming home on time, or the boss calling you in for an unexpected meeting.

We are plagued by the frightening thoughts of our child being abducted, or the boss handing out our notice. When thinking about these situations using a calm sense of rationality, we could come to more likely conclusions such as the noise actually being a falling object, our child's bus only running late and the boss just wanting to give you a new task relating to work.

These situations are usually resolved in due time and we commonly enter a quick state of relief due to these frightening possibilities not becoming a reality. However, this is where anxiety can cripple us. Anxiety can seemingly force us into believing irrational scenarios (such as those mentioned above) even when we aren't faced with such scenarios. We can begin to fabricate our own scenarios with our own devised, variable outcomes for that certain situation. Let me explain further.

Say for example we were suffering from a persistent headache, but we *didn't* suffer from an anxiety problem. Our thought spread may look similar to this:

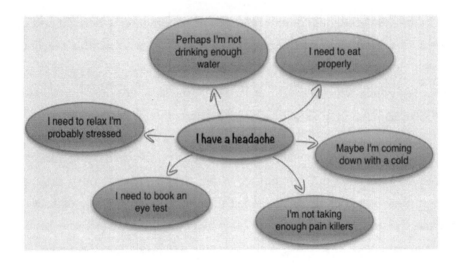

Each of the thought conclusions represents a common form of rationale with at least one of them likely to be the answer or 'solution'. Using a balanced sense of rationale we can almost conclude that the cause of the headache is down to one of the thoughts/possibilities above. Everyone experiences headaches at some point and they are almost always no cause for immediate concern.

Now let us look at how a high state of anxiety can affect a person's use of rationale using the same headache scenario used above. Below is another thought spread representing how anxiety can cause us to believe in the scariest but unlikeliest of scenarios:

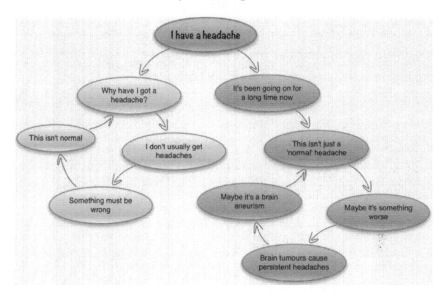

Look at how anxiety can distort and change the thinking process when dealing with a scenario. The first headache scenario shows how a calm sense of rational thinking can help us find a quick conclusion to a situation. However the one above represents when something as simple as a headache can quickly develop into an anxious problem. The headache in this situation has now turned into a worry and thus has caused *more* anxiety.

The thinking process in the second diagram actually creates a twofold problem. When we are anxious we look to attach reasoning to the anxiety to help us understand why we feel the way we do. The more extreme the anxiety, then the more extreme the worst case scenario appears to be.

Using the previous example, the headache is assumed to be something that's potentially dangerous and frightening - a worst case scenario. Not only has anxiety lead us to this scary and irrational conclusion, but we have also added a further worry to an already stressed mind and body. This can be applied to any situation or worry including suffering from anxiety itself.

It's interesting to see what happens when we put anxiety itself as the variable in our scenario. Instead of using the headache as our scenario try and replace it with 'adrenaline' and explore the possibilities.

# PART 2

## Anxiety Symptoms Explained

This section of the book provides explanations to the symptoms that are associated with having an ongoing anxiety condition. Here you will find itemised an encyclopedic-style symptoms list, along with explanations as to why and how these symptoms can be caused by anxiety. There will undoubtedly be symptoms that will not relate to you, but I certainly recommend that you to read through them all so that you're well equipped if they ever occur in the future.

The information provided here derives from a combination of personal experience and observational research about the topic of anxiety, but is in no way official medical print or to be prioritised over the opinion of a health professional. Having said this, I am extremely confident in stating that each symptom found here all have direct links with anxiety and the likelihood of the symptoms being caused or aggravated by anxiety is, in my opinion, unquestionable.

The symptoms list at the start of this book separates the symptoms into two lists – the **psychological symptoms** and the **physical symptoms**. In this part of the book I have ordered the symptoms list starting with the most commonly occurring symptoms, then moving towards the more obscure symptoms.

You will find that the explanations to certain symptoms will sound familiar or relate to other listed symptoms. This is due to anxiety and its symptoms all being linked together, which in itself is positive in terms of simplifying everything and assuming we have an anxiety problem - much like the *anxiety umbrella*.

# 1. Derealisation / Detachment / 'Feeling weird'

**What?** This occurs in almost everyone who experiences excessive anxiety and panic. Derealisation occurs when our reality and surroundings feel and appear distorted and we become highly aware that we feel 'different' from our usual selves. It's common for many sufferers to feel very lucid at times of derealisation and almost entirely detached from their surroundings. Many have described it as feeling like they are uncomfortably floating, or as if they're existing in a room in third person.

You could be, for example, in a certain place that's very familiar to you, but the natural feelings and recognition associated with the place are missing. Feelings of vertigo, light headedness and tunnel vision are also common when identifying an episode of derealisation. It's important to understand that episodes of derealisation can be responsible for a large number of panic attacks and can often act as the trigger, due to it seemingly creeping up from nowhere and being immediately misunderstood.

People often find it extremely difficult to relax at times of derealisation and often fall into the trap of trying to over-think a way out of it. Over time derealisation can outweigh feelings of normality and can actually present itself for a longer periods of time compared to being in a 'normal', settled state. This gives the victim a false projection of reality, causing all sorts of problems and swaying a person's perception of the world around them. Feelings of derealisation are completely harmless and will pass with time, patience and a change in behaviour habits.

**Why?** Derealisation occurs as a result of a stressful routine and an accumulation of negative thoughts and behaviours. It can also appear as the result of trauma. It's a sign that the body's nervous system is hypersensitive and that the body is also currently working on a chemical imbalance by releasing all sorts of chemicals into the blood stream.

Feeling lucid and detached from your surroundings is also an indicator that there is an abnormal amount of adrenaline floating around your system. High amounts of adrenaline cause us to become hypersensitive and it temporarily alters our nervous system - putting us on high alert for signs of a 'problem' or danger, causing us to intricately analyse ourselves and our surroundings.

During episodes of high or abnormally flowing adrenaline, our bodies change in response to the chemical. Our peripheral vision shuts down, our breathing alters and our ability to focus becomes difficult. Feeling detached from our surroundings - particularly when we don't know *why* we feel detached - can be extremely frightening for those who find it hard to deal with a lack of control. However the feelings inevitably subside as the adrenal gland will either stop releasing as much adrenaline or will eventually exhaust itself.

# 2. Unexplainable Fear / Fear of going 'insane'

**What?** Fear is an emotion that becomes embedded within us as we grow up and is also part of our make up as human beings. However, when worry and fear become irrational to the point where it is debilitating to our lives, then it becomes an obvious symptom related to an anxiety problem. An anxiety condition usually presents itself with episodes of mild to extreme bouts of unexplainable fear. This is due to the body dealing with doses of adrenaline and cortisol which are usually released at times we're not expecting.

Unfortunately, we sometimes try to make sense of this fear by attaching our own fabricated reasons and thoughts to it. Mild fears such as going to the shops, or suffering from a persistent headache, become exaggerated fears which can be moulded to explain why we are feeling so anxious. Going to the shops suddenly becomes too dangerous, and the headache is the sign of a brain tumour. Furthermore, this unexplainable fear has been the reason why so many people have taken unnecessary trips to the emergency department, or rang for the emergency services because they are convinced they're having a heart attack or that they're going insane. We try to make sense of the fear by attaching a worst case scenario to explain it. This all ties in with 3.3 in Part 1 - *Rationality and Worst Case Scenarios.*

This fear causes us to take up all sorts of irregular behaviours. This includes pacing around a room, finding it difficult to relax, scanning our body and environment for 'problems' and trying to work out *why* we feel the way we do. The fear can also channel into a person's fear of panic attacks.

The fear has always been present since the evolution of the anxiety problem, but because the prospect of having a panic attack is so frightening we can become stuck in the loop of peaking anxiety - *worrying* about having another panic attack. This is another example of applying reasons to attach to the fear as a means of making sense of it.

**Why?** As explained above, the intense presence of fear is due to an imbalance within the body and the presence of fear-inducing chemicals such as adrenaline. The imbalance occurs as a result of a poor thought routine, which confuses the brain into thinking when and where is the best time to become ready to activate the 'fight or flight' response. This would explain why fear can suddenly overwhelm us from nowhere, or that we become unusually fearful of a circumstance that wouldn't usually warrant such a response.

Fear is one of the main barriers that can hinder a positive change when tackling anxiety. Although I and many other anxiety victims hated feeling anxious on a daily basis; I unfortunately felt a degree of comfort knowing that anxiety was the only constant in my life. I felt that if I tried to change, or do things differently, than I would make my 'condition' worse. Take note that this is completely irrational and borders on the absurd. Fear prevents you from doing things that you have learned to be dangerous. Changing who you are - for the better and for a more positive life - is not a dangerous task.

# 3. Hyperventilating / 'I'm not getting enough oxygen'

**What?** The feeling where breathing becomes an added effort and all of our attention is suddenly focused on our breathing. This can be misconceived as feeling like we're not getting enough oxygen, or it can create a panic reaction because we question why we're breathing so abnormally. Irregular breathing usually occurs when we feel panicky and anxious, but can also happen when we're feeling physically encumbered by things such as stomach bloating or tiredness.

**Why?** Almost every anxiety sufferer has been concerned about breathing at some point when living with the condition. When we are anxious our heart rate usually increases, so to compensate for this we breathe in more oxygen. Throughout the day we begin to shallow breathe because the anxiety has caused us to take in more oxygen than what's required. However, many mistake this natural shallow breathing as the feeling that we're not getting enough oxygen, so we then begin to breathe in more – and we begin to hyperventilate. The body can't produce the carbon dioxide it needs to get rid of in time so we can find ourselves hyperventilating for quite a while.

During a panic attack it's very common for someone to hyperventilate and it can often prolong the panic attack. That's why so much importance is placed on breathing when dealing with anxiety and panic. Shallow breathing can also be responsible for other anxiety symptoms, such as: heart palpitations, chest pains, feeling lightheaded and dizzy. It can also alter the way we think and provide difficulty when trying to focus.

The short term benefits of controlling our breathing are helpful and that's why it's promoted so widely, but I personally feel that too much importance is placed on trying to 'control' the breathing because it can apply heavy pressure on the anxiety sufferer. When we are anxious it is common to be very self-aware/hypersensitive to any changes or abnormalities that occur in our bodies. I feel that focusing on abnormal breathing often creates a negative effect, as it can often lead to panic and hyperventilation. Although it causes other symptoms, shallow breathing isn't particularly dangerous and you'll actually find that it 'disappears' when you deal with the core of the problem. It's an anxiety problem, not a breathing problem.

# 4. Heart Palpitations / Flutters / 'Skipping a beat'

**What?** I have found that almost every anxiety sufferer - including myself at the time of writing this book - at some point experiences sensations and differences in the rhythm of the heart. Heart palpitations are a sudden fast beating of the heart that seems to occur either unexpectedly, after some form of physical exertion, or triggered by a negative thought. They can happen as frequently as every day, every week or just once in every while. Heart palpitations can also present themselves as a fluttering sensation in the chest and sternum area, and also the feeling that your heart has 'skipped a beat'.

Heart palpitations can happen to anyone and usually pass unnoticed to the majority of people. However, they can intensify and increase in frequency when they're considered a problem by the common anxiety sufferer. The process of worrying about heart palpitations creates a catch 22 situation; the more we worry about the palpitations specifically, then the more frequently they seem to occur.

The link between worrying specifically about the palpitations and the frequency of them isn't mutually inclusive, but when we do persistently worry about them we are easily lead into states of hyperawareness because we fear them occurring again. We succeed in noticing and living through every noticeable change in the rhythm of the heart - even those that are natural and occur every day in almost everybody. This is called being left in a state of apprehension, which causes our bodies to become tense and we're ultimately left in an irrational state of hypersensitivity waiting for the next palpation/flutter/skipping a beat to happen again.

**Why?** There are various reasons why differences in the rhythm of the heart can occur. Heart palpitations, chest flutters and temporary irregular beating are found to be very common with anxiety and are almost certainly not a sign of a serious heart condition (please see a health professional if you have doubts). There are many causes that trigger a heart palpitation, not all of which can be identified prior to a palpitation occurring. Some of the most common causes are down to:

1.) **A surge of released adrenaline**
2.) **An electrolyte imbalance**
3.) **Hormonal changes**
4.) **Too much oxygen**
5.) **Physical exertion**
6.) **Change and fluctuations in blood pressure**
7.) **Anxious thoughts**
8.) **Diet factors e.g. caffeine, sugar intake, nicotine**
9.) **Dehydration**
10.) **Periods / Menstrual cycle**
11.) **Medication**

I used to suffer from palpitations on a daily basis and over time they began to calm down when I began to focus on my initial reaction to them. I taught myself that they weren't going to cause me any harm and that although they were scary, it was ultimately down to factors associated with my anxiety that were causing them. To help further my aim I changed my diet, quit smoking, cut out caffeine and drank more water.

I notably found through my research and the collaborative views of others that all of the causes listed above are all linked in some way to being anxious - either physically or psychologically. Firstly, stress and anxiety often cause us to make drastic changes to our diet. It's common for an anxiety sufferer to search for 'escapes', or temporary relief through things such as alcohol, fatty comfort foods and smoking. We are perhaps lead to eating drastically more or considerably less and our water intake maybe differs from our usual consumption. Diet factors, stress, medication and dehydration can all make differences to our blood pressure, which in turn causes further noticeable changes in our bodies including changes in the rhythm of the heart.

Our electrolyte levels are altered by the physical symptoms of anxiety, physical exertion, lack of nutrients from our diet and dehydration. We lose electrolytes through our sweat - either through exercise or sweating when we're anxious or panicking. An electrolyte imbalance is often a cause for palpitations to occur, which can be fixed with an improved diet and adequate hydration. Then of course the most common cause of heart palpitations in anxiety sufferers are the surges of adrenaline that seem to occur at any time of the day. An adrenal and hormonal imbalance directly affects the heart rate, but is actually harmless and becomes less frequent when the sufferer comes to terms with the condition.

Chest flutters aren't always linked with the heart and are often misinterpreted as the heart 'fluttering' or beating quickly. Acid reflux, trapped wind, I.B.S and indigestion often release gastrointestinal gases and create excess stomach acid, which can apply pressure to the chest and sternum area causing a 'fluttering' affect. This will be explained further later on under *Irritable Bowel Syndrome*. Flutters can also be mistaken for spasms in the chest muscles, which are another very common symptom of anxiety.

## 5. Chest Pains

**What?** Anxiety can often cause the victim to feel various pains that can occur in and across the chest area. It's important to note that these pains can alter in the way they present. The types of pains include sensations of stabbing, cramping, aches (dull to severe), shooting pains and pain that's dependant on position of the body and the current state of breathing.

Unfortunately, the pains are often mistaken for something worse than what they actually are and because they can vary in terms of the type of pain, the location on the chest and the time of day they can strike, they can often cause the anxiety victim to assume the worst about them. For example: a stabbing pain across the chest is assumed to be a heart attack, an ache is automatically acute angina and chest pressure suddenly becomes a lung problem.

Chest pains often act as the trigger for setting off panic attacks too - particularly when they occur alongside a heart palpitation (although they are usually mutually exclusive).

**Why?** There are several reasons why chest pains occur as a result of an anxiety problem. The first and primarily the most common reason is muscle tension. Anxiety and adrenaline cause our muscles to tense up - even when we think we're not tense - and a lot of the tension centres on certain points of the body. These areas are mainly the chest, back, shoulders and abdomen.

When we're dealing with a lot of adrenaline, our muscles tense up to provide an outlet for it all. Our core upper torso muscles seem to 'scrunch up' like a sponge - acting as the body's way of dealing with the adrenaline. As a result this causes all sorts of muscles to be expanded and contracted almost entirely against our will. Throughout the day our muscles can do this - they can happen throughout daily life such as work, chores and social occasions.

The muscle tensing process is harmless in the long term, however in the short term all the scrunching, tensing and contracting will cause all sorts of pain that can differ from muscle to muscle. Good posture and muscle stretching is the key to alleviating the pain that tension causes, as well as taking any focus away from the pain being something irrational (a sign of something serious and unlikely).

Chest pains are also commonly linked with Irritable Bowel Syndrome, indigestion and excess stomach gases. Our digestion cycle can be affected by anxiety, due to our body focusing on dealing with the adrenaline and other bodily chemicals that are released during periods of high anxiety. The stomach can often produce excessive acid and gases which push up against the chest causing pressure against the sternum and chest muscles. An observation of the digestive cycle is usually required to identify this as the cause, as well as noting what you've eaten prior to chest pains occurring.

# 6. Hypersensitivity / Body checking

**What?** During periods of anxiety we may become prone to scanning our bodies for signs of an anomaly or trying to find something that's wrong. When we become confused about the way we feel - particularly when anxiety and panic strikes unexpectedly - we can immediately turn the attention to ourselves to find the cause or reasoning to why we feel so differently.

Hypersensitivity is when we find ourselves in a state of self observation; we are scanning our bodies to try and find problems to *justify* the intense feeling of fear we are experiencing. For example, we may think that an odd pain we experience is a sign of something serious, perhaps we become irrationally fearful of something in our environment, or a sense of *derealisation* indicates that we're potentially going insane.

Unfortunately, hypersensitivity seems to work hand in hand with anxiety. When we are anxious and dealing with lots of adrenaline we may - without even acknowledging it - attach odd reasoning to why we feel the way we do.

For example, when we are anxious our breathing alters (shortness of breath) and our heart often palpitates. Our reasoning may tell us that the shortness of breath and the rapid heartbeat are the culprits for this anxiety, when in fact it is quite the opposite.

If you find yourself constantly scanning your body then I'm afraid that you're already anxious! It is common for most people to experience palpitations and differences in breathing and often passes unnoticed. However, when we are hypersensitive, we often 'clock on' to every twinge and difference we spot within us which just adds to the worry pile. The breathing becomes a serious issue and the heart palpitation is suddenly something severe.

**Why?** Hypersensitivity occurs as a direct result of adrenaline being released into the system, but is unfortunately intensified through repetitive habit. When our body activates our 'fight or flight' response, we immediately enter a mode of hyperawareness– something that's handy in times of danger and is part of our genetic makeup. However, when an anxious episode strikes the same process happens, except that confusion often follows because there is often no identifiable cause/danger in front of us. The hyperawareness can then become channeled into hypersensitivity and we begin to analyse ourselves.

After all, if there's no danger in front of us, or an easy explanation, then it must be our bodies that are the cause of the problem.

Over time self-analysing or body checking can turn into a bad habit. We begin to search for things that simply are not there. The simple process of body checking causes a lot of unnecessary stress for the body to handle.

# 7. Panic Attacks

**What?** A panic attack is when an intense feeling of fear, dread, loss of control and entrapment overwhelm a person. Accompanying these feelings are thoughts of an imminent disaster, impending doom and even the fear of sudden death. A panic attack is often unexplainable and can appear to strike without an identifiable trigger. The physical symptoms that can occur alongside this are feelings of detachment, vertigo, dizziness, light-headedness, shortness of breath, muscular pain and various vision impairments. Panic attacks can occur infrequently (once in a while) or several times a day.

Panic attacks are often responsible for 'unnecessary' trips to the hospital and can often 'mask' themselves as a heart attack, stroke or mental 'breakdown'. The most prominent effect of a panic attack is its unbelievable ability to make somebody believe the most irrational and unlikeliest of scenarios and outcomes. These scenarios include the belief of sudden death against all logic (I'm having a heart attack!), the unlikely explanation of a symptom or the feeling that all existence will end almost immediately. Sufferers can often find the experience so terrifying that they fear it will happen again. This unfortunately leads to many being stuck in the 'loop of peaking anxiety' which was mentioned in Part 1.

**Why?** A panic attack happens when the body releases a large amount of unexpected adrenaline into the bloodstream. Adrenaline can cause all sorts of changes both physically and mentally – the most prominent change being the stimulation of our nervous system.

If we're unprepared or 'caught off guard' by a newly released dump of adrenaline, then it could be expected of us to panic about this sudden change. The panic comes from the confusion about what is happening, alongside believing that you cannot cope. Adrenaline actually causes our minds to race and be filled with all sorts of thoughts and conclusions as to *why* we're panicking and *why* we're feeling strange.

This would explain why so many people are convinced that they're having a heart attack, or that they're going insane, or that they have an incurable condition and so on. It is the adrenaline that affects our rationality during these periods of panic, thus causing them to turn into prolonged *panic attacks.*

These panic attacks don't last forever because the adrenal gland finally becomes exhausted and cannot release any further adrenaline. Our nervous systems also settle in due time. The reader should take comfort in the fact that a panic attack cannot last forever because of this and the feeling of normality will return. It's what you do next that determines the severity, intensity and frequency of any potential panic attacks in the future.

## 8. Fear of having a Panic Attack

**What?** Fearing a panic attack itself is perhaps a clearer symptom of anxiety than any other. Many who have experienced the horrendous experience of a panic attack are in fact so terrified of one happening again that they spend the majority of their time anticipating another one. This is called being left in a state of apprehension - similar to what I explained when discussing heart palpitations above. It's actually a simplistic loop that many people have experienced or have become stuck in. This state is often exclusive to people who have been diagnosed with panic disorder.

**Why?** The experience of having a panic attack is often a terrifying ordeal for the individual who lives through it. Anyone who's experienced a panic attack would obviously wish to never have one again, but for some people the fear is so prominent that they spend the majority of their time self-analysing as a means to apprehend one if it strikes.

The process of doing this is self destructive as it adds to a person's overall anxiety and creates a stress that hinders daily life. Ultimately, a panic attack is a temporary loss of control and it's this loss of control that drives us to try and control every aspect of anxious thoughts and behaviours.

# 9. Nausea (Feeling Sick) / Frequent Urination / Diarrhoea

**What?** Nausea is the feeling where it feels like we need to vomit. Frequent urination usually coincides with the need to empty our bowels on a frequent basis. Basically we feel we need to go to the toilet a lot. Stools are found to have a liquid consistency and we may pass wind more frequently than usual.

**Why?** It's common knowledge that when we're anxious or nervous about something, we often feel 'woozy' or that we may be sick. Perhaps this could happen before a job interview, a public event or awaiting important news about something. Alongside this we may find ourselves going to the toilet a lot more than usual.

Basically, all that's happening is an offshoot of the body's 'fight or flight' response. When the body prepares itself for imminent danger, it tries to relieve pressure on the organs by releasing things inside the body such as water, food, gases and stomach acid. The brain tries to pressure the stomach into pushing out all of the digesting food, acid and gases. Our bowels are rushed into action to empty everything it contains - that's why we often get diarrhoea or poor quality stools. Furthermore, the bladder begins to work overtime to try to rid the body of any excess water.

# 10. Fear of Sudden Death

**What?** This is the feeling of an imminent disaster or death - even against all logic and rationale. This could be a thought that branches from a panic attack or feeling overwhelmed.

**Why?** When anxiety is high, so are our levels of adrenaline. High amounts of adrenaline place us firmly in 'fight or flight' mode, which alters the way we view our surroundings and prepares us for worst case scenarios. Death is arguably the foundation of any worst case scenario, so it's not surprising that many with anxiety feel extra sensitive when it comes to mortality. Death is *the* worst case scenario and sometimes acts as the most compatible reasoning to a very intense bout of anxiety and panic.

# 11. Headaches

**What?** Obviously most of us will know of and experienced many headaches in our lifetime. However, it is important to be aware that headaches come in many forms and for a variety of different reasons - this is particularly important when relating headaches to anxiety.

A head ache can present itself as a <u>mild to severe aching</u> sensation, <u>short stabbing pains</u> across the scalp and temple, a <u>stretching/throbbing</u> sensation across the head and pain that seems to <u>emanate from beneath the skull</u>. The duration of a headache can vary as well with some headaches merely spanning an afternoon, whereas others can last for more than two weeks plus (my longest headache lasted over a month). The headaches can present as constant, they can alter in severity, they can 'come and go' and they can vary in response to painkillers.

**Why?** Headaches can arise because of factors such as dehydration, eye strain, malnutrition, sun stroke, stress and as a symptom of another illness such as hay fever or the common cold. These name just some of the many reasons why headaches can occur. In relation to anxiety, headaches mainly occur because of <u>stress</u>, muscle tension and <u>poor posture</u>. Stress causes our bodies to seize up and adrenaline causes our muscles to tense up. To cater for this we often and quite unknowingly alter our posture to accommodate for all of this muscle tension.

Over time poor posture - whether standing or sitting - causes the muscles on our scalp, neck and shoulders to become weathered and stretched. Our muscles are expanding and contracting all the time and the added effort of stretching *against* our poor posture causes aches and pains all over the head area. Imagine your scalp and shoulders being made of thin rubber and that rubber stretching as your posture curves inwards. Stretching and posture alteration is the key to alleviating head pains caused by muscle tension.

Dehydration and poor appetite are also contributing factors to a headache. The body cries out for nutrients and water and when this need isn't met it causes a stress on the body – this can cause a headache. Furthermore, a lack of sleep (insomnia) and a poor sleeping pattern can easily cause headaches, especially when we find ourselves overly tired.

# 12. Agoraphobia - 'The fear of going outside'

**What?** It is very common for a lot of people with an anxiety problem to fear going outside. Agoraphobia is, more often than not, found to be directly linked with an anxiety problem due to the irrational nature of the fear itself. To the agoraphobic person the outside world becomes 'out of bounds', due to it being perceived as too open, too dangerous, believing they may not cope if taken away from their current surroundings or the fear of how the general public may perceive them.

When I was dealing with the peak of my anxiety, I recall hardly ever leaving the house for the fear that I may have a panic attack, or that I simply just would not cope. I also feared what my local community would think of me, which only intensified my underlying fear of going insane.

**Why?** Agoraphobia is the result of anxiety and all of the symptoms and thought associations that come with it. Racing thoughts, unexplainable fear, irrational thinking and hypersensitivity can make you perceive the world as an overwhelming place, when in fact it is the combination of your body's chemical imbalance (adrenaline) and the irrational associations and beliefs that you hold about the world outside.

Some people - particularly those who *suffer* from agoraphobia - believe that it is the outside world that's responsible for their anxious thoughts and not the other way around. This is simply not the case. We as anxiety sufferers can become agoraphobic due to the power of association we place on our surroundings, especially when anxiety is at it's highest and we feel the safest in our own homes. What you must realise is that anxiety prevents you from thinking rationally, so it comes down to willpower to convince yourself that the outside world is no less of a place than the inside of the home.

# 13. Irritable Bowel Syndrome (I.B.S)

**What?** Irritable Bowel Syndrome (also known as spastic colon) is surprisingly common in people who have experienced a prolonged anxiety problem. Symptoms of I.B.S include stomach bloating, acid reflux, trapped wind, constipation, diarrhoea, stomach pains, sore rectum and gastrointestinal discomfort. It can also cause notable variations in the types of bowel movements that we have and the frequency in which they occur. Some people can observe which foods tend to 'trigger' the I.B.S, with some of the most common being foods that contain spice, gluten, wheat, lactose, fat and high amounts of sugar (it varies for each individual). It is not uncommon for people who have undergone large amounts of stress to develop intolerances to the food listed above.

**Why?** Anxiety affects the body's chemistry, which in turn affects things such as the immune system, hormone production and the digestive cycle. I don't know the full biological process of how anxiety affects the digestive tract, but there is officialised medical print to confirm the direct link between the two. What is known is that anxiety can cause changes to our blood pressure, metabolism and also creates excessive amounts of muscle tension - particularly in the abdomen. This leaves no doubt as to the impact anxiety can have on abdominal area, which contains the fuelling engine for our bodies.

# 14. Abdominal Pains

**What?** Abdominal pains are pains that occur across the abdomen and can vary in the way that they present. These include <u>feeling sore</u>, <u>stretching sensations</u>, <u>stabbing</u>, <u>shooting pains</u>, <u>cramping</u> and <u>general aching</u>. The location of these pains can alter in their position on the abdomen and can also fluctuate in intensity. It is possible for a lot of these pains to be happening at once and can happen at any time of the day.

**Why?** There are two common reasons why abdominal pains can occur when linked with an anxiety condition: the first being that the pain is an offshoot symptom of Irritable Bowel Syndrome (as explained above). The second reason and perhaps the most common is down to muscle tension and posture. Muscle tension is responsible for all types of pains due to anxiety causing us to expand and contract our muscles intensely and excessively. Adrenaline causes our muscles to tense up - even against our will - so if we don't stretch and relax accordingly, we feel the consequences through erratic and varied pain. Poor posture also intensifies this muscle tension, especially when we are hunched and our shoulders are too far forward. Stretching, posture change and movement are the key to alleviating the pains.

# 15. Tiredness / Lethargy / Exhaustion

**What?** This is the feeling of being overly tired or lethargic in comparison to a 'usual' state or degree of expectation for the time of day. Furthermore, you could be experiencing frequent states of exhaustion that have taken up a commonplace role in day to day life.

**Why?** Simply living with an anxiety condition is tiring enough, as it causes the body to work hard all of the time. Anxiety can cause the body to do all sorts of 'unnecessary' overtime in the form of maintaining a fast heart rate, taking in too much oxygen, a distorted digestive cycle, muscle tension, processing racing thoughts, dealing with copious amounts of adrenaline and so on. Furthermore, anxiety affects sleeping patterns and the overall quality of sleep, which over time accumulates and presents itself in the form of chronic lethargy. Although troubling, tiredness is not a cause for concern and unfortunately is inevitable when anxiety is a constant.

# 16. Excessive Perspiration (Sweating)

**What?** Sweating is a normal bodily function that's intended to cool us down when our body temperature is high. However, when it becomes excessive, or occurs more frequently than usual, it usually has a direct link with anxiety. Sweating can occur when we are anxious, after strenuous exercise, after eating certain foods or whilst we are in a hot climate. It can also occur for no apparent reason - this is usually exclusive to the anxiety sufferer.

**Why?** When we are anxious our body temperature naturally rises due to the heart and body having to work harder. Furthermore, anxiety is also the trigger of the 'fight or flight' response and during this the body tries to push out any excess fluids through urination and sweating. When anxiety becomes a prominent feature in our lives, so do the symptoms that can occur with it - excessive perspiration being one of them. Drinking lots of water and working on the core of the problem is the solution to this.

# 17. Muscle Pains & Spasms

**What?** Muscle pains and spasms can occur all over the body, but are particularly prominent in the chest, abdomen, back and shoulder areas. A spasm is the sensation of a muscle quickly tensing and expanding against our will and can occur with or without pain. Odd twinges and pains can occur in our muscles too and they can happen in almost any muscle in our bodies.

**Why?** As explained before, anxiety and adrenaline causes muscle tension all over the body, which is adjunct with the body's 'fight or flight' response. It is a perfectly normal bodily reaction, but over time the constant tensing of muscles can take its toll, with the muscles becoming overly strained, inflamed and overused.

Muscle spasms are also linked to dehydration and a poor diet. Spasms and pains are very common in the chest and abdominal areas and are often mistaken for something worse. The chest, abdomen and shoulders often take most of the tension, thus making them prime spots for pains and spasms.

## 18. Dehydration / Dry Mouth / Feeling Thirsty

**What?** Dehydration occurs when the normal water content of your body is reduced due to releasing more water than it's taking in. Symptoms of this can include: <u>experiencing dry mouth</u>, <u>feeling thirsty</u>, feeling lightheaded, <u>dry lips</u>, nausea, lethargy and passing urine less frequently or in lesser amounts. Dehydration can also lead to feeling unusual or detached from our surroundings (derealisation). Dehydration can also trigger panic attacks as it raises the heart rate and can make us feel dizzy and unstable.

**Why?** A water imbalance (dehydration) can occur due to a poor appetite and bad habits, where we don't take in enough water, we excessively perspire, frequently urinate, alter our breathing and pass watery stools. When we are anxious, we actually need a lot more water than usual to compensate for the loss of water.

Dry mouth can be recurrent due to not only the water imbalance, but can be attributed to nasal obstruction and excess stomach acid. Stomach acid has a low PH and kills off some of the bacteria in our mouths that keep our mouth hydrated and healthy. Drinking lots of water and a healthy diet are key to alleviating dehydration and dry mouth.

# 19. Eye Floaters

**What?** Eye floaters present themselves as strange 'blobs' or cell-like shapes that float across the eye-line regardless of where we are looking. They are small pieces of debris that can vary in size and can look like black shadowy dots, fluffy dots, long narrow strands and noose-like cells. These 'floaters' get their name because they float around the eye's vitreous humour - a jelly-like substance within the eye ball.

**Why?** Floaters are very common in a lot of people and are usually not the sign of a serious eye condition. Floaters are the debris floating around in our vitreous humour and also the shadows that they cast onto the retina. In relation to anxiety, it is unknown if there is a direct link between eye floaters and suffering from an anxiety condition.

What is known is that anxiety causes victims to be hyperaware and hypersensitive of themselves and their surroundings. Eye floaters usually pass unnoticed by many or aren't regarded to be dangerous, however, when we are anxious we can often fixate ourselves on the floaters and assume the worst about their presence.

If they do become excessive it would be wise to seek a doctor's or optician's opinion, but in most cases they are harmless. I still have the floaters in my eyes but they pass unnoticed unless I feel anxious. Anxiety causes our peripheral vision to shut down and our vision to alter its focus thus making the floaters more apparent.

# 20. Difficulty Relaxing / Inability to Keep Still

**What?** Anxiety often acts as a stumbling block when it comes to relaxing or trying to 'wind down'. It can cause the simplest of relaxed activities to become laboured and effortful. Activities such as reading, watching television, writing, knitting etc, can feel strenuous and unnatural.

We often worry when we aren't able to enjoy the things we usually partake in, which can add to the overall anxiety. Moreover, a lot of activities and chores require focus and the ability to remain still. Anxiety can cause us to worry to the point where we fidget or even pace the room in a desperate attempt to provide an outlet or to 'keep it together'.

**Why?** It's very difficult to relax and focus when we are anxious because of the chemical imbalance within our bodies. Adrenaline causes us to be 'on edge' as part of the body's 'fight or flight' response. It causes our minds to be flooded with copious amounts of thoughts, as well as causing physical changes to how we operate. The 'fight or flight' response is designed as a defence mechanism for when we sense danger. Unfortunately, an anxiety condition can confuse the brain when it comes to defining literal danger and imaginative danger. It becomes very difficult to relax or 'switch off' as the chemicals in our body are prepared for danger instead of allowing us to relax.

# 21. Rib Pains / Pressure under the Ribs

**What?** Anxiety can often be the cause for rib pains and pressure under the rib cage area. The pains can vary and can present themselves as a dull ache, sharp pains, pain in the muscles between each rib and general discomfort under the rib area. Like many other symptoms, rib pain is often misconceived as something worse than it actually is.

**Why?** There are two main causes for rib pain in relation to anxiety. The first is muscle tension and the effects of consistent muscle contraction and poor posture. The top of the abdomen, including the rib muscles, is a prime spot for muscle tension caused by anxiety. Furthermore, anxiety causes our posture to change and we can often hunch up and push our shoulders forward, which intensifies the effect of the contracting chest and rib muscles.

The second and just as common reason can be put down to Irritable Bowel Syndrome and indigestion. Indigestion, trapped wind and a poor digestive cycle can cause excess gas and stomach acid to build up in the stomach. Gravity has little effect on gases, so they naturally rise and become trapped in areas of the stomach causing a slow build up. The top of the stomach expands to cater for the excess gas and acid, which in turn causes the stomach muscles to press against the rib cage. This is responsible for a lot of rib and chest related pain.

# 22. Search Engine Obsession

**What?** We can often turn to the internet for the answers to life's questions. We can do this by using various search engines that provide us with a list of results/answers after a quick click of a button. With regards to anxiety, unhealthy search engine use is when we obsessively trawl search engines and websites for the answer to our anxiety problems.

We can often spend hours clicking, scrolling and reading mass amounts of information that usually serves to be counterproductive when trying to alleviate stress and worry.

**Why?** The internet has rapidly become the first and fastest point of reference for obtaining information. When we feel anxious or panicky, we often want a quick solution or fix to the problem. Unfortunately, we can often fall victim to believing that search engines have the immediate answer.

Search engines are designed to chronologically list websites that are 'best tailored' to the search that you requested. This is defined by how popular a website is, the information contained within the website or how much a web developer has paid to place their website high on the search ranking list. This leads to all sorts of websites being thrown up by search engines. It can often be hard to define which websites are set up with good intentions and those which are set up solely for profit.

I would personally advise anyone to limit their internet searching, as too much information can become overwhelming and an anxious mind is susceptible to the negatives that such information might provide. Anxiety causes us to reach irrational conclusions and I have found that relating to what we could define as 'medical print' from sleek, professional websites causes more bad than good. Go to your General Practitioner for a diagnosis.

## 23. Ringing in the ears / Tinnitus

**What?** Tinnitus presents as a constant or broken up ringing in the ears. It can vary in pitch, volume, frequency and can often still be heard when the ears are covered. It is known to cause discomfort, insomnia, dizziness, lightheadedness and panic.

**Why?** Tinnitus can often be permanent as a result of damage to the internal ear. However, with regards to anxiety, I have found that tinnitus has not remained permanent with those who have managed to battle and overcome their anxiety.

# Anxiety: Panicking about Panic

There are many factors that cause tinnitus, with anxiety being a major cause. If you're experiencing it don't panic. Instead, just focus on your anxious thoughts and the symptoms will subside. Please visit your doctor if you have any concerns.

# PART 3

Now that we've covered the 'ins and outs' of anxiety and the array of symptoms that accompany it, we can now move on to making the next positive steps to actually overcoming it - just like I did many moons ago. You may or may not realise this, but just by reading up to this point of the book you have already taken a giant step towards a 'recovery', even if it doesn't feel like it yet.

The core foundation when tackling anxiety and perhaps when dealing with almost any difficult problem in life, is to form a strong understanding of it. When we simplify a problem, it inevitably becomes easier to tackle and eventually fades to the point where it isn't actually deemed a problem at all. When we *understand* that anxiety isn't this dangerous and complex condition we initially perceive it to be, we can begin to strip it down, piece by piece, until its true harmless face is revealed.

This part of the book will provide straight up advice and steps as to what to do next to ease the persistent fear that anxiety causes and return to normality. Remember that you're not isolated with this problem. It's alarmingly common. Even when the strangest of things happen and you're stuck in a bit of a strange place, always remember that the feelings will eventually reside and that 'you' will return to normality.

# 3.1 It's Just Anxiety

## Stop trying to work your feelings out!

Seriously, just stop. As anxiety sufferers we often become worried, confused and frustrated at the continuous and sometimes unrelenting nature of our condition. As we have learnt, the very process of worrying about our condition, as well as trying to 'work it out', only brings negative attention to the problem and acts in a way that's counterproductive when trying to alleviate all of our problems.

Just by merely thinking about anxiety produces a negative effect on the mind and body. It releases adrenaline and sets us off on the same negative thought paths where we can find ourselves back at square one - worrying why we feel the way we do and scanning ourselves for signs of disaster.

Many of us - including myself - find ourselves stuck in the same repetitive thought patterns, where we try to work out why we feel the way we do and in a lot of cases looking for that miraculous thought/epiphany where we feel that one thought can conquer all of our worries and symptoms. Unfortunately, this 'miracle thought' is impossible to accomplish, as anxiety is the result of poor routine and a biological imbalance within the body. I'm sorry to say this but one thought cannot fix your problems and the only way out of a problem caused by poor routine is to trade it in for a fresh, healthier routine and a positive mental outlook.

Now this may seem easier said than done - particularly when anxiety appears to cripple us and any task seems like a physical and emotional mountain to climb. I used to think simple tasks such as posting a letter or going to the shops was out of my reach. It's also common thinking that the prospects of change, doing something different or taking ourselves out of our comfort zones is just an action that sets us up for a fall. Thoughts revolving around negative outcomes like 'not being able to cope' and fearing panic attacks often act as a stumbling block when actually getting out and establishing a new routine.

In order to take your second step towards overcoming anxiety (the first being the establishment of your understanding), you need to **immediately implement a change in your behavioural patterns**. Stop trying to work it out because, quite frankly, there isn't anything to work out! You know what anxiety is, where it has come from and what happens within your body when anxiety and panic strikes. You need to snap out of the routine that only promotes anxiety and irrational thinking and start a new one. It is a scary prospect but it doesn't take long for your positive actions to dampen the severity of your scary thoughts.

Now you may be questioning why and how this would help at all. Let me explain using a common scenario:

"Rebecca has been suffering with generalised anxiety and panic disorder for around 3 years. She finds it very difficult to leave the house and as a result of this lost her job a year ago. She lives on her own and hasn't the confidence to get back in touch with her friends, or establish new relationships due to fear of leaving the house and struggling with severe social anxiety. She wishes she could feel like she 'used to', or a time where like how she felt *before* the anxiety started.

Almost every day she wakes up hoping to feel 'normal' again, but is immediately disappointed when she finds that she still feels the same and that there are still odd things happening to her body. Her first thought when she wakes up is *'Do I feel ok today?'*. When she doesn't feel the way she wants to she starts to panic. She panics because yet again everything doesn't feel normal and that she feels like she's living with an incurable, psychological condition. The panic then defines her world around her and sways any decisions and motivation that may have existed with the freshness of waking up from sleep.

Her thoughts then turn on herself. She begins to body scan. *'Why have I still got this headache?'*, *'this pain is still here'*, *'something is seriously wrong with me'*, *'I feel like I'm going insane!'* she often thinks. She then starts to try and rationalize and apply logic to give herself hope: *'I'll work this out! It'll be something deep and complex but once I've found the answer I'll be ok again!'*

Rebecca proceeds to pace around her house and exhaust herself. Every day she waits for the feelings to pass, or for that miracle thought to enter her head. Sometimes, when she feels ok, she reasons with herself that the anxiety has passed. This is until the symptoms of anxiety crop up again. Her chest flutters, she feels lightheaded, her breathing changes and her mind is flooded with undesirable thoughts. She's back to square one. *'What's wrong with me?'"*

It's obvious from this scenario that Rebecca has been confined to her own negative thought patterns and has fallen victim to abiding by her own sense of irrationality. Rebecca is constantly anxious and has found herself stuck in the 'loop of peaking anxiety'. Rebecca believes that her problems will go away by abiding by the same anxiety-dictated routine and thought patterns that revolve around worry. She thinks that simply by waiting and trying to 'think her way out' of it she will eventually get to where she wants. She has been suffering for 3 years.

What Rebecca needs to do - this applies to all of us - is to change her behaviours both physically and mentally from the moment she wakes up. She needs to realise that there is nothing to work out - she simply has anxiety. Instead of waking up and thinking *'Am I ok today?'*, she needs to think, *'Ok well I've had anxiety and these symptoms for a while now. I accept this and I'm going to do something productive today regardless of how I feel'*.

We need to realise that our bodies take time to recover from the symptoms anxiety can produce. Pains, aches, derealisation, an imbalance of adrenaline and all of the other symptoms can take a while to subside, but they *will* subside given the chance. So for now just ignore them. Rebecca needs to ignore how she feels because she *knows* she has anxiety and a plethora of things 'wrong' with her.

With that out of the way, we can now begin to change our behavioural habits. Positive rationalisation tells us that the outside is no more of a danger than sitting inside. Setting goals that challenge our fears, such as going outside, begins the process of rewiring the default thought process of our brains.

The more we rely on emotional crutches, such as the walls of our homes, then the more we'll end up back at the beginning. The more we keep our minds occupied on tasks, hobbies, fun activities and socialising, then the less we keep our minds on bad thought patterns, such as dwelling on the anxiety or working out our problems. Believe me this works.

Set yourself a goal no matter how simple it may seem. If *you* find it a scary and difficult task then I suggest you bravely undertake it. For me it was doing the simple things like catching the bus to work, going to the supermarket or going for a short walk. You'll find that nothing bad happens despite your feelings telling you otherwise. You have to ignore your gut on this one and rely on willpower. There's no use sitting in thinking away your problems.

This is the first step: stop working it out. In Part 1 we discussed grouping all of our symptoms and problems into one manageable problem. Using the anxiety umbrella, we can put all of our excessive and irrational worries to one side and concentrate on dealing with it as one manageable problem. This includes psychological worries about our mental health, as well as the physical worries that come with anxiety, such as derealisation, heart palpitations, chest pains, tiredness, headaches, panic attacks etc.

Excessive worry is just anxiety. That's it.

# Lose the *'What If?'* because it's just anxiety.

It's a normal part of the human thinking process to contemplate different types of outcomes to any given situation. In *Rationality and Worst Case Scenarios* we covered several types of irrational conclusions that our mind can lead us to when we're in a state of anxiety. What we have learned is that anxiety causes us to distort our thinking to the point where we simply focus on the frightening possibilities and less on the harmless, more likely outcomes.

As you'll know these frightening possibilities, that manifest themselves as thoughts, can easily be dwelled upon and can often dictate our plans and actions in our daily lives. Anxiety almost always stops us from what we want or 'used' to do - making it a crippling stumbling block when it comes to living the life that we want to.

Both consciously and subconsciously, a life consumed by anxiety can lead us to question situations with the fore-fronting question *'What if?'*. Applying the *'What if?'* question to scenarios in life isn't necessarily a bad thing, with it being vital in terms of keeping us safe and avoiding any potential, negative ramifications in a given situation. When *'What If?'* is applied to justify irrational fears however, then it becomes a problem.

We can apply *'What If?'* in common situations such as approaching a blind bend when driving, opting to walk home through a well lit area or perhaps thinking twice when bringing up a sensitive topic of conversation in a group full of people. This use of logic can help keep us safe and avoid any upsetting consequences that could occur, such as avoiding a car crash or offending somebody for example.

However, excessive anxiety, which often leads to hypersensitivity and hyperawareness, can create an abundance of *'What if?'* in our lives, which can lead us to apply the question to normal, every day things. We can start to question our normal daily actions and the *'What if?'* starts to take centre stage when we begin to apply our logic. Normal every day activities, such as going outside, going to social occasions or even taking the journey to work, can suddenly be perceived as a dangerous task that would be best left avoided, due to fear of a panic attack or something awful happening.

Furthermore, from a hypochondriac perspective, we can also begin to question the symptoms that occur with anxiety. We can begin to look at feeling different, experiencing bodily changes and all of the other symptoms that come with anxiety as something that's a 'worst case scenario'. For example: a head ache becomes a brain tumour, a palpitation becomes a heart defect or a sense of derealisation is the first sign of insanity.

Let us look at some rational and irrational *What If's* to clarify:

# Rational 'What If' Scenarios

- ❖ *"I really want to stay for another drink"* - What if I'm too drunk to get up for work?
- ❖ *"I can't be bothered to go back for my bike helmet"* - What if I have an accident?
- ❖ *"I'll risk not wearing a jacket today"* - What if it rains?
- ❖ *"I want to make a joke about this subject"* - What if I offend my colleague?
- ❖ *"I think that stray dog looks friendly"* - What if it suddenly attacks?

# Irrational 'What If' Scenarios

- ❖ *"I need to go and get the grocery shopping"* - What if something bad happens outside?
- ❖ *"I must get the busy train to work"* - What if I have a panic attack?
- ❖ *"My heart keeps pounding and skipping beats"* - What if I have a heart attack?
- ❖ *"My friend has invited me to a party"* - What if they think badly of me?
- ❖ *"Everything suddenly feels different"* - What if I'm going insane?
- ❖ *"The doctor says there's nothing wrong with me"* - What if I've been misdiagnosed?

We all use irrationality to shape and strengthen our use of rational thinking and logic. Therefore, quite hypocritically, the process of irrational thinking is in actual fact a *rational* process. It only becomes a problem when the irrational thought becomes our conclusion - a walk to the shops becoming too dangerous for example.

This is where the next and debatably most difficult step arises in overcoming anxiety. <u>You have to lose the *'What if?'*</u>. In order to lose them, you firstly need to do something that, at first sounds simple, but actually takes a lot of willpower to apply. You need to identify the irrational *'What if?'*'s and simply ignore them. In order to identify and ignore them, you need to dig deep and use your own sense of positive rationalisation and apply it to the scenarios where you think anxiety is stopping you from doing the things you should or need to be doing.

When I was struggling at the peak of my anxiety, I wouldn't even leave the house. I feared what the outside world would think of me if I suddenly became overwhelmed with anxiety or had a panic attack. One day I decided to lose the *'What if?'* and actually used positive logic to weigh up the possible outcomes of leaving the house. I decided I needed to go food shopping and in doing so ignored all the feelings, thoughts and emotions I was going through in order to do it.

I managed to make it to the supermarket and almost had a panic attack in the vegetable aisle. I was so close to turning around and running home, but I stuck at it and *imagined* the pride I'd feel if I completed the shopping. I did eventually complete the shopping and the sense of achievement I felt when I got home actually helped ease the anxiety I was feeling. I was scared of the *possibility* of something bad happening, not the reality. I also realised that my home was my 'safe place' and that I was using it as an emotional crutch. Going to the supermarket helped me to temporarily live without this.

Positive rationalisation is a fancy named term that's the equivalent of saying *'It's just anxiety'* out loud. Lose the *'What if?'*'s and blame everything that scares you on anxiety. Pop up your anxiety umbrellas and let them shield you from the monsoon of irrationality that rains upon you. Get out there and have a go.

# It really is 'just anxiety'

In section 1.1 we looked at grouping all of the thoughts, fears and symptoms together. We labeled them as one problem and I explained about the use of the *Anxiety Umbrella*. A good way to distinguish between a 'normal' symptom and that of a symptom of anxiety, is to look at it comparatively to a time where you once felt ok.  What also helps is that sometimes, deep down, we know that our thinking can become quite absurd, so we can use positive rationalisation to identify what thoughts are normal and what thoughts are caused by the anxiety.

I cannot stress enough the benefits of labeling our symptoms and fears as 'anxiety'. We know that anxiety will eventually ease and what helps is that an onslaught of several symptoms at one time can be found to be manageable, with the knowledge that they're only caused by one thing! For example, you could be suffering from a prolonged headache, experiencing a lack of appetite, worrying about chest pains and perhaps being scared to attend a social event. These are several different symptoms to contend with, but they don't need to be dealt with individually. <u>They are all just anxiety</u>. They will all pass in due time and if they don't go away then you're more than likely refusing to accept that it's just anxiety.

Here are some diagrams consisting of common symptoms where anxiety is directly involved:

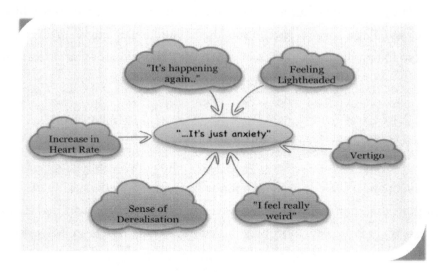

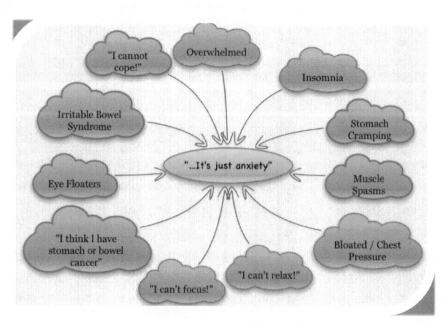

As you can see from the examples above, there are several listed anxiety symptoms which all point to one common cause - anxiety itself. Each symptom on their own can be found to be scary or discomforting and it doesn't take a lot for the anxiety sufferer to imagine how overwhelming it feels for these symptoms to be happening all at once. Anxiety can be blamed for many other feelings and symptoms - most of which are listed in **Part 2** of this book.

As you can see in the second scenario, there seem to be several symptoms happening at the same time, but they are all linked to one cause. I and many others have found that we've had many more symptoms happening at once or recurring frequently. The only thing that linked them all was anxiety.

Anxiety creates so much stress on the body and we must realise that the symptoms can come in abundance. Put it all down to anxiety and you'll quickly find that it becomes a manageable problem to contend with.

# There's nothing 'wrong' with you

Suffering with anxiety, regardless of how long you have put up with the condition, should not be feared as there isn't actually anything wrong with you. This is arguably a bold statement to announce, given all the turmoil and emotional distress anxiety can cause. However, a major key to recovery is to realise that anxiety itself is not an illness; it is definitely not dangerous and can be fixed through the uses of a strong understanding, a change in behavioural habits and becoming a reflective practitioner when it comes to tracking and analysing our thoughts.

Anxiety is a condition that develops over time as a result of poor mental routine and solidified behavioural habits. Note that the key word in that statement is the word 'condition'. A condition is something that can be changed and altered and is in no way represented as something permanent. Simply by stating that you have an anxiety condition means that the condition you're currently in can be changed. You are not stuck with this forever and change can be implemented immediately.

Anxiety is not an illness simply because it's a bodily process that occurs naturally. Think about it; we wouldn't deem breathing, our digestive cycle, sweating and sleeping as a problem or illness - it's simply something that our body does naturally. Anxiety should be placed into the same bracket as this because all that's happening within our body is completely natural. It's an overuse of our 'fight or flight' response. We're simply dealing with the effects of living with an erratic adrenal gland and over stimulated nerves. The abnormal feelings and symptoms that come with it are merely a matter of perception. Let me explain further:

The most difficult part of dealing with the anxiety is undoubtedly the *fear* it triggers within us. We fear that of definitive change, but quite ironically most of us wish that we could change back to how we felt before the anxiety started. We've learned that the feeling of fear comes predominantly from the chemicals that are released into our bodies, mostly adrenaline and cortisol, as well as any emotional recognition attached to a given thought.

The fear - caused by this chemical imbalance - acts as the main factor when we mould our perception of the anxiety. We are quick to assume that anxiety is this terrifying and crippling burden that has been thrust upon us, instead of simply acknowledging that it's a naturally occurring bodily process that's as harmless as the hiccups or trapped wind.

As a result of habit, we consciously and subconsciously *tell* ourselves to be anxious and actually self-trigger the fight or flight response in our bodies. We fall into the same thought habits by dwelling on the same daily worries, thus giving us the same daily anxious response.

This needs to change.

It is not the fault of our adrenal gland and it is not the fault of our bodies. It is *your* thoughts that are the cause! Begin to change your thought patterns and you'll begin to change your anxiety for the better.

# The Power of Thought

Your body reacts to all types of thoughts. Your body constantly reacts to these thoughts by releasing chemicals such as adrenaline, thus causing your body's natural balance to be constantly disturbed. Never underestimate the power of a thought and what it can do to your body!

Take a moment to think deeply about how much a thought can massively affect the body. It's something that we already know and have acknowledged on a subconscious level, but it's essential that we use this knowledge, as it acts as one of the key weapons when tackling and understanding anxiety. Let us look at a few examples:

❖ Try to think of something that excites you or remember a time where you felt overwhelmed with excitement. E.G. *a holiday, a gig, a first date, seeing a close friend, a new episode of your favourite TV program, an adventure, a hobby etc.*

It is the <u>thought</u> that excites you because you're imagining being in a desirable position. You know that you're going to enjoy the exciting event/occasion, because you've either done it previously, or are eagerly anticipating a new positive experience. Take note of the surroundings when these exciting thoughts occur.

You could be at work, walking down the street, doing the ironing or being just about anywhere. More often than not the surroundings would have little to do with you dwelling on these positive thoughts, because you're thinking about what is planned for the future (of course your surroundings can trigger the thought if it reminds you of something). Note how the body can react to what you see in your imagination, as well as what you can see in front of you.

❖ Try to think of something that scares you. E.G. *a rollercoaster, spiders, enclosed spaces, fear of losing a loved one, open water, dying.*

Even in the safe comfort of your own space, these thoughts can affect the body. When I comprehend the thought of a spider crawling across my face, scuba diving in an underwater cavern or perhaps thinking that I'm going insane, it does cause me some minor discomfort.

When dwelling on this thought I can safely say that I'd be in no mood to engage in one of life's laborious activities. What about those feelings of dread before a job interview? Or an upcoming meeting with somebody or something that frightens you? Once again these thoughts can have little to do with what's around you, with only your surroundings serving as a reminder. Simply by imagining myself in these undesirable positions has caused my body to react in its own way. Can you see what I'm puzzling together here?

The point I'm putting across is that it is <u>thoughts</u> that can affect the body. Anxious thoughts are part of being human, but excessive worry and negative thoughts can and *will* affect the balance of the body. When anxiety is largely understood this imbalance is easily rectified, however when we find ourselves in a poor mental state - crippled by fear and racing thoughts - it becomes harder to think clearly and rationally. Just say to yourself, *"I will think about this when the anxiety and the adrenaline has passed. I'm too anxious to think clearly at the moment."*

Bear this in mind the next time you find yourself dwelling on your anxiety or any scary thought. The thoughts can affect the body and it's no wonder we find ourselves in such negative states if we're constantly feeding ourselves negative thoughts. Just remember that negative thoughts create negative emotions.

We often dwell on what scares us as a way of coping with the issue, even if the event has happened or may happen in the future. It provides us with a false sense of control about an issue that scares us. Just let anxiety run its course without providing it with any more fuel. If you can achieve this then you're well on your way to beating anxiety and demonstrating a strong understanding of it.

## Anxiety should not be feared

Sounding like I'm highlighting the obvious, anxiety often evokes the feeling of fear. However, anxiety itself should not be feared. If we fear anxiety and panic occurring then we simply bring it on ourselves. Just by fearing anxiety, we evoke exactly the same emotion we feel when we are anxious! We need to <u>constantly remind ourselves that anxiety cannot hurt us</u>. Just remember that anxiety is just another name for the body's 'fight or flight' response, which is constantly irritated and triggered by worry and fear.

Let's just think about it. If a fluffy bunny rabbit came hopping towards you in the street, your body wouldn't suddenly change and release adrenaline because you do not fear it. You *know* the rabbit is coming but your body doesn't enter 'fight or flight' mode because there is no dangerous association that your mind has formed of the bunny rabbit.

Now let's switch the bunny rabbit with a rabid dog and re-run the same scenario. This time the dog comes towards us and our 'fight or flight' mode does kick in. Anxiety starts because we are worried about the danger in front of us - rapidly foraging through scenarios in our minds about what the rabid dog could do to us. This 'fight or flight' mode is there to protect us and kick start our bodies in the face of danger. Unlike the bunny rabbit, our mind associates the rabid dog as a danger.

It all boils down to perception. If you perceive feeling the symptoms of anxiety as a danger, then you'll spiral into a pit of worry that takes a long time to climb out of. Every time that you start to feel different, whether it be experiencing derealisation, obsessing on a thought or feeling something physical, then this is a time to test yourself. It's all about your reaction.

Treat feeling anxious as the bunny rabbit instead of the rabid dog. There's no need to add heaps of worry onto what the body is currently experiencing. The feeling will pass and will actually present itself less and less severely the more you train yourself to just tolerate it. You'll find that your anxious episodes become less frequent and also less intense. This is explained further in the following sections.

# 3.2 Change the bad habits. Re-wire your brain.

## Stop over-thinking and 'Body checking'

It's ever so common for the average anxiety sufferer to over-think their problems and to try to 'think their way out of it'. We have learned that this is merely counterproductive and actually acts as a catalyst for the anxiety to kick-start. When we think about anxiety and try to 'think it away', we are actually adding another worry onto all of the other worries that we may currently be dealing with.

We also bring a large amount of attention to the anxiety which, for our hypersensitive bodies, puts us on high alert for change and danger. We don't want these anxious feelings to be present, so we're constantly on lookout for any sign of it disappearing, as well as trying to spot signs of it progressing or 'getting worse'.

Furthermore, when we are unaware or forget that anxiety has grasped hold of us, we sometimes look inwards for signs of something wrong. Many anxiety sufferers turn to scanning the body in order to attach reasoning for why they feel the way that they do. This is often the case when adrenaline is pumping through our bodies and that we have failed to acknowledge that we're currently in an anxious state.

Many people suddenly put immeasurable amounts of focus on something that they wouldn't normally deem so troublesome. This focus could be on many things, such as a change in breathing, a chest flutter, chest pains, dizziness, vertigo, derealisation, irritable bowel syndrome, ringing in the ears and so on.

What makes this deplorable is that we can cause ourselves to worry further about the symptoms we are focusing on, which in turn can cause the overall effect of the symptom to become worse or increase in intensity. For example:

Anxiety and worrying can cause heart palpitations. Worrying about the palpitations causes anxiety. With increased anxiety come more frequent palpitations, which are perceived as being 'worse', or more intense due to the extreme focus that's placed on them. You can summarise it as a two-way process. Anxiety causes palpitations. Palpitations cause anxiety. Take a look at this diagram for a clear picture:

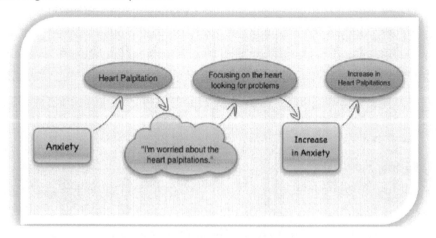

This isn't just the case for heart palpitations. Over-thinking and focusing on other symptoms unfortunately causes the same effect. For example, worrying about a headache causes stress and tension, which can actually make it worse. Worrying about chest pains causes us to tense up, causing any current chest pain to increase in intensity. Worrying about I.B.S disrupts our digestive cycle, thus making that a further problem too. This also applies to sweating, feeling sick, tinnitus, various muscle pains etc.

The very process of worrying about the anxiety actually makes the anxiety present itself with increased intensity. This is something that we have covered during the earlier stages of this book. When we over-think and try to 'think our way out' of anxiety, we actually bring attention to the fact that it's there – affecting our lives. We become hypersensitive to it, thus making it feel more intense. The anxiety takes a more prominent stage in life, therefore making it feel like a bigger problem than it actually is.

Of course worrying doesn't make every symptom worse. If you're worried about dying, going insane or something that lies out of your control, then your anxiety remains at its 'capped limit'. Remember that anxiety cannot kill you and that the thought processes of your mind have little to no effect on the outside world. Anxiety reaches a limit - with that limit being the undesirable emergence of a panic attack.

Stop placing so much focus on your symptoms and I guarantee they will disappear, or drastically reduce over a relatively short amount of time. Acknowledge when they are reducing and make the link between your new thought routine and the reduction in anxiety. Stop over-thinking and body checking. In order to make this task easier, you need to keep your mind occupied in a healthy way.

# Do what you'd usually do, or try something new!

Keeping your mind occupied is undoubtedly one of the best things to do when snapping out of a bad routine crammed full of bad habits. In a lot of cases, in particular relating to my battle with anxiety, the anxiety sufferer is often found with a lot of time on their hands to aimlessly think about all sorts of issues and the complexities of life. Or in a lot of cases, particularly if you're a person who has a natural tendency to worry, we think about things that trouble us. We often do this because it acts as a coping mechanism in case the issues we worry about ever strike, or we treat it as a life puzzle for our minds to form an answer to.

The process of doing this isn't necessarily a bad thing. However, if we're already stuck with an anxiety condition then this 'thinking time' is often put to bad use. It's ever so common for many to use this time to dwell upon the anxiety and the symptoms that it causes. We know from the previous section, and throughout this book, that thinking and focusing attention on the anxiety is a counterproductive process. We bring attention to the issue, which actually makes it more of a problem.

Anxiety, quite sadly, stops many from doing what they would usually do in their everyday lives. Activities, hobbies, socialising and daily requirements, such as work and chores, can easily become a no-go zone for many, which is why anxiety often leads to depression. Depression kills our motivation and any positive associations we have formed with what we used to deem as fun or interesting - making it even harder for the anxiety sufferer to motivate themselves to break out of their negative routine.

This is where I lay down the next piece of advice for you and I think that it's essential that you follow it. Simply do what you would usually do. If you feel that the positive association you had with your old life has been all but lost then simply try something new. As an anxiety sufferer you need to re-wire your brain into a new, positive routine - something that does not happen overnight, but gets incredibly easier over a short amount of time.

Doing what you'd usually do doesn't mean acting out your current anxiety fuelled routine; it means partaking in something that you once recognised as necessary for your daily life. You may have to cast your mind back way into the past for this, depending on how long you've been hampered by anxiety. This includes doing things which you once enjoyed, or just acted out without a second thought. I remember enjoying taking the busy train to the beach, filing away paper work for my job and spending time with all of my friends. These things I did without question, but became disillusioned with during my time with anxiety.

Wake up and imagine what you would do with your day if you didn't have the anxiety and do it anyway. The effects of a poor thought routine will try to stop you on your journey, but remember to just ignore them. Thoughts cannot harm you.

# Change your reaction and you'll change the anxiety

To begin re-wiring your brain in order to cope with or rid yourself of anxiety, you'll need to change your behavioural habits. The best way to do this is to firstly monitor how you react to the dumps of adrenaline that are released into your system, or in other words, how you react to when you suddenly become overwhelmed by anxiety or panic.

When I reached a saturation point during my struggle with anxiety, I literally hit a point where I tried not to care anymore. It was a motivation dictated by anger. This was an anger deriving from the predicament I was in. I had reached the end of my 'tether' and was disgusted at how my life was being dictated by this anxiety. I decided that I would do what I would usually do, regardless of how I felt, just to regain a sense of control in a life where I felt control was scarce.

So I took it upon myself to live out a 'normal' daily schedule and simply use willpower to ignore any changes or symptoms that anxiety threw at me. Every time I experienced an episode of derealisation, panic, chest pains and breathlessness - I just carried on. I continued doing what I set out to do and was in no way going to let anxiety prevent me from doing it. I did the house chores, I watched a movie, I went to visit friends and I walked the dog.

Now the symptoms of anxiety did crop up, but by simply trying to ignore them and keeping my mind focused, they actually didn't feel as intense as they usually did. Be under no illusion - I still felt pretty terrible and continuously on high alert, but I did notice an incremental difference in the severity of my anxious feelings. I changed my reaction to the anxiety by simply continuing what I was doing. My reaction changed. I was beginning to re-wire my brain.

The symptoms still felt horrible, but what I noticed is that by keeping my mind occupied and focused on something else, the anxiety only felt at about 60% of the intensity than what it would usually feel like if I was confined to the walls of the house - focusing on my problems.

I'd caught on to something quite remarkable.

I decided to experiment with this approach, as it took the sting out of the anxious feelings I was experiencing on a daily basis. The anxiety was still there, but it didn't feel crippling anymore; it was more like a debilitating feeling that I could push through. I thought that if keeping my mind occupied helped ease the anxiety a little, then maybe it could have an accumulative effect in terms of continuously easing the anxiety. I thought that maybe the more I kept myself busy, then the less my anxiety would be present. If anxiety ever struck, then I would force my reaction to be minimal and keep my focus away from concentrating on the symptoms.

This is actually something that works so well that you can actually notice a significant difference in a matter of days. There are stages of the day where you can actually feel 'normal' and, to some degree, content with the situation.

My reaction to the anxiety was always under the spotlight.

I tried my absolute best to keep a low level reaction when anxiety struck and, quite incredibly, I noticed the frequency and intensity of the anxious episodes slowly decrease.

You must work on your reaction to the anxiety - particularly when panic strikes. Use positive rationalisation to assume that there is nothing wrong. Just assume that it's the feeling of anxiety and continue with whatever you were doing, or channel your focus on something productive. I have worked with many people using this plan and they will tell you that this approach works. It takes time and energy but the results happen quicker than you think. You will surprise yourself.

# Give yourself something to look forward to

Further to changing your reaction to the anxiety, you can also take a step forward by facilitating the adrenaline that pumps through your system. This book goes some way to explain to you that adrenaline and other bodily chemicals, such as cortisol, are one of the prime factors when it comes to the *feeling* of being anxious. However, adrenaline and fear don't always run parallel with each other. We mustn't forget that adrenaline forms a part of other positive feelings that we experience - the feeling of excitement for example.

When we feel excited, this feeling is stimulated by various chemicals – including adrenaline. Further to this, adrenaline helps us to enjoy things such as exercise, competitive activities, sport, sex and responding when put under pressure. As explained before, adrenaline also forms the main part of our 'fight or flight' response, which is a vital bodily function which aids us in keeping us safe and helps us to mould our perception of what we deem safe and dangerous.

A key skill required to gain back a sense of control over your anxiety is to try and channel your thoughts down a more positive thought path. You can do this by thinking and focusing on something that you're really looking forward to and excited at the prospect of doing. This actually helps in more ways than one, because it helps take the 'edge' off of any depression (or helps prevent it) and also eases the load on the adrenal gland and nervous system.

By veering your thought path and focusing on something you can enjoy, you are channeling the adrenaline into doing something that it is useful for.

Try and focus on something that actually lifts your mood.

Common examples include looking forward to a holiday, attending an exciting event, a new episode of a TV show, a visit from a relative, a day out or even pay day.

Anxiety, along with depression, is often described as possessing an inability to see a positive future. By trying to focus on something that you enjoy - no matter what it is - you are actually taking a step in a positive direction - regardless of the enthusiasm being there or not. So give your body a positive outlet for the adrenaline by thinking of something that's exciting or that you're looking forward to.

# Don't associate feeling anxious to future events

When we think of doing anything under the influence of anxiety, our perception and emotional recognition with what we're thinking about can often become skewed. Anxiety often leads us to thinking that simple tasks are actually monumental in terms of using energy and draining us emotionally. Furthermore, when we try to think at a time when our bodies are dealing with a chemical imbalance, this can often lead to the feeling of fear being attached to activities and events that we're thinking about doing in the future.

In this part of the book I have explained that you should do what you would usually do in a situation, or try something new, as a way of breaking out of an anxious routine. I explained that this requires willpower and conjuring the ability to ignore anxiety when it skews your thoughts and tries to distract your attention with its symptoms. When anxiety skews your thoughts, it can extinguish any enthusiasm you may have for planning positive things to do in the future. Take these common scenarios for example:

❖ "I'm feeling horribly anxious and I don't think I'll make the birthday party this weekend."

- ❖ "I don't want to visit the doctor. I'm going to hear something awful."
- ❖ "The last thing I want to do is go to the gym."
- ❖ "I don't think I'll cope with visiting relatives next week."
- ❖ "I'm in no state to go to work tomorrow."
- ❖ "I haven't got the energy to do the house work today."

These statements all have one thing in common. They are all a pre-emptive assumption about a future emotional state. The fact is that we don't know how we'll feel in the future, but as anxiety sufferers we have become used to the ever present, predictable nature of anxiety and the symptoms that accompany it. We unfortunately *assume* what we'll feel like in the future.

Yes, anxiety can and will drain our enthusiasm and lead us into depressive states. But the key here is to not make plans based on a current state of mind or present emotion. Yes, you'll probably be anxious at the time of making a plan, but like I explained before, you should just do it anyway. You don't know how you'll feel in a years time, a weeks time, an hours time or even a minutes time.

By second guessing your emotional state, you're actually *choosing* what mindset to be in when the event or scenario arises. Instead of pre-empting how you'll feel, try and take a gamble and see if it pays off. Let's take those presumptions from above and remould them using positive rationalisation:

- ❖ "I realise that I'm anxious, but maybe the party this weekend will take my mind off of it. I may find that I actually have fun!"
- ❖ "I probably will be anxious at the doctors, but I know it's just anxiety and I'll feel better afterwards after some closure."
- ❖ "I'm unmotivated for the gym, but maybe it'll provide an outlet for all of this adrenaline."

- ❖ "I'm sure I'll be in a better mood to visit Grandma next week. I'll plan it anyway."
- ❖ "I'm anxious tonight but after some sleep I'll be alright for work. I'll do it anyway and show this anxiety no attention."
- ❖ "I can keep my mind occupied by doing some household tasks. I'm sure that when I start I'll get into it."

Don't let a current anxious state dictate what you plan to do for the future. In fact you shouldn't let it get in the way of what you want to do now. Use positive rationalisation and willpower and refrain from giving your anxiety any undeserved attention.

# Stop researching your symptoms on the internet!

As anxiety sufferers, we can forgive ourselves for trying to find the answers to a problem that we're confused and worried about. Unfortunately, many of us turn to the internet for our answers. Quite ironically - and in contrast to one of the main ways this book can be discovered - trawling the internet usually serves to fuel anxiety and panic instead of alleviating it.

You must remember that when you type your symptoms into a search engine, you are entering data into an almost entirely pure market space. Almost the entire internet is a capitalist fuelled world, where people buy and sell products, services and information. When typing anything into a search engine, you are presented by these products and services with the top search results represented by the websites who are the most popular, or who are the highest bidders. This is the same market of which I sell this book.

You'll be aware that the world around us presents us with a variety of advertising and selling techniques usually revolving around the concept of false 'need' instead of 'want'. Unfortunately, when typing health matters into a search engine, we are presented with a plethora of websites offering to sell us products, medicines, cures and methods to 'help' us with our problem. Unfortunately, one of the most commonly used and easiest methods in marketing is the practice of 'scaremongering' people and using them as the target market.

As an anxiety sufferer, it's a very common behaviour to type in our symptoms into search engines as a measure of providing relief from our panic and the feeling of being isolated. Sadly, this is where many businesses have formed a target market. We as anxiety sufferers are in need of help and many online businesses see this as an opportunity to sell their products, where the legitimacy of them is always under scrutiny.

Referring back to *Anxiety and Worst Case Scenarios,* these websites serve to use scaremongering tactics to make us aware of these worst case scenarios. Typing isolated common symptoms of anxiety such as palpitations, headaches, dizziness and panic, causes our screens to be flooded with cleverly, sugar-coated scaremongering techniques aimed at trying to persuade us to buy products, or scaring us into a sense of insecurity where we're at risk of purchasing something due to our state of vulnerability.

You may have found that symptoms such as heart palpitations are directly linked to a heart defect. Chest pains are almost certainly a sign of angina and chest problems. There's a good chance that your headaches are the sign of a brain tumour and dizziness is probably related to a life-threatening blood pressure problem. Although there are plausible links to these extreme cases, probability tells us they are simply the uncommon, worst case scenario with the odds being further heightened by the fact that you have anxiety.

Furthermore, websites such as forums, blogs and chat rooms include people who thrive off of the fear they can create. Of course I find the vast majority of forum members and bloggers are found to be perceptibly kind and opinionated. However, when we're anxious we are easily drawn to the negative scenarios due to the underlying fear and adrenaline that drives us to find a solution to our problems. People can be quick to share an extreme story about someone they know or have heard about. Usually, stories that are way out of the norm draw immediate interest. This interest then represents itself in its search engine ranking.

For example, *Blogger A* writes about how a woman he once knew collapsed and died after having a headache at work. Or how *Forum Member 1* explained how his friend once had a heart palpitation leading to his heart exploding. These types of stories are prominent at the top of search engines as anything out of the norm gains large amounts of interest.

Stop using search engines to find the answers to your symptoms, unless you use a logical and rational approach. The internet isn't all full of tripe like that mentioned above, but just be careful when deciphering legitimate information and unethical sales pitches.

# If you're looking for something then you'll find it

When we're confused about an anxious state we find ourselves in, we often look for a reason to attach to the unexplained anxiety. We can often fall into bad habits as explained before, such as body checking, focusing on harmless symptoms, or even using our imaginations to conjure irrational dangers in our outside environment.

There are also many other things that we seem to point the finger of blame towards. Such blame can revolve around our personal and social lives, as well as us questioning our own mental health.

Anxiety sufferers - including myself at one point- often make it part of their common daily routine to knowingly or unknowingly search for blame or a reason as to why they feel the way they do. This behaviour can easily become obsessive, but often disguises itself in a normal daily routine. When we obsess, particularly when it relates to anxiety, we almost always think we have the right conclusion in our minds, but we're just searching for clarification or evidence to justify it.

For example, when we feel anxious, we can often find ourselves trying to 'think our way out' of anxiety. When this approach doesn't seem to work, we can easily conclude that something must be wrong with our minds. However, we've already had our minds made up that something is wrong, because why else would we try to think our way out of anxiety? We've already assumed that something is wrong because why would we do something so irrational as to search for a miracle thought to rid us of anxiety?

This type of obsessive thought can be applied to when we try to analyse our symptoms too. Take heart palpitations for example. If we convince ourselves that something is wrong with our heart, we can often find ourselves obsessing and focusing intensely on the rhythm and beating of the heart. Almost every person's heart beats out of a predictive rhythm at least once a day and it passes unnoticed. However, to the obsessive anxiety sufferer it becomes highly noticeable and immediately a problem. The anxiety sufferer assumes there's something wrong with the heart and so sets out to find a reason to justify the assumption. They find the reason to attach to the way they feel without realising that all they were feeling was just anxiety.

This can be applied to many other symptoms: stomach pains, headaches, dizziness, chest pains, derealisation - to name a few. As explained in *Stop Over-Thinking and Body checking,* this process is counterproductive and actually deflects our focus from the actual problem. In a nutshell, obsessing about something that frightens you, with regards to anxiety, means you'll more than likely find what you're looking for.

# 3.3 Helpful Anxiety Advice

## Score your anxiety levels

When you begin to notice differences in your anxiety levels, particularly when they become less intense, you can begin to give them a rating in terms of intensity and how anxious you feel at a given time. This really helps when it comes to looking at your anxiety comparatively and you can use it to measure and acknowledge how you're progressing. It's also helpful for target setting and acts as a motivational tool to try something that we might initially feel uncomfortable with.

I began to score my anxiety when I could safely deem that the majority of my usual week felt 'normal' - where the feeling of abnormal anxiety was outweighed by the feeling of content. This is not to say that I completely rid myself of anxiety and as a matter of fact it still creeps up on me now and then and still to this present day. I still use this scoring method as it acts as a reminder of how far I have come and I couldn't recommend it any stronger than I recommend this entire book.

Below is the anxiety scoring method table. This method can be altered and tailored for the individual. I personally use this one. Nowadays my anxiety usually averages at around a score of 2 or 3.

# Anxiety Scoring Method:-

**1 - 2 = Low level anxiety.** No different from the average person. Usually represented by a feeling of anticipation or the feeling of impatience. Feeling stresses from a to-do list or a daily routine.

**3 - 6 = Moderate Anxiety.** Aware that there's a generous amount of adrenaline in the body. Feeling fairly uncomfortable and unable to relax. Intrusive thoughts and a significant effort to ignore irrational thoughts. Able to acknowledge that the feeling will pass.

**7 - 9 = High Anxiety.** Symptoms prominent particularly depersonalisation. Breathless and aware of symptoms such as derealisation, feelings of dread, palpitations, dizziness, vertigo and any other that has been obsessed about. Unable to think clearly or operate at a normal level both physically and emotionally. Scanning for signs of disaster. No motivation except for escape.

**10 = Panic Attack.** The feeling of complete derealisation, depersonalisation, confusion and imminent disaster. Panic symptoms aplenty. The feeling of no escape and impending doom. Common symptoms include a pounding chest, breathlessness, inability to focus and balance. Complete breakdown in attachment to surroundings.

The scoring method is exactly how it presents. Instead of saying to yourself, *"Oh no it's the anxiety again,"* you can actually score your anxiety and look at it comparatively. One day you may feel a bit uneasy, so instead of just folding to the assumption that it's anxiety, you could actually say to yourself, *"well I feel quite uneasy and my anxiety feels at around a 4."* You can begin to look at anxiety as measurable.

By scoring your anxiety, you're actually establishing a preventative process where you've acknowledged how you currently feel and can immediately start to ignore certain thoughts and symptoms that arise. After a certain amount of time you could then re-score your anxiety levels to see if they've come down. You'll find - more often than not - that this happens.

Comparative scoring can also be helpful in situations that you may find difficult. Common examples include: being in a crowded place, travelling, social situations, health matters and even just being outside of the home. You can begin to take encouragement when you notice the overall or average levels of your anxiety decreasing.

Of course not every occasion will provide a positive result because anxiety can vary in intensity. It is important not to take any notice or attach any importance to this if it ever occurs. Just keep going and your overall anxiety average will slowly decrease.

## Lose the Emotional Crutches

In any stressful life it's common for someone to rely on little escapes and emotional crutches in order to get through the day. Common escapes include: smoking, drinking, recreational drugs, medication, computer games, over sleeping etc. I'm not here to discuss the pros and cons of doing such things, but I do feel these things can act as a stumbling block when they're completely relied upon as *emotional* escapes.

Common sayings such as *'I can't give up smoking because it would make everything worse'*, *'I'll always need this medication'*, *'I need a drink to ease the nerves'*, *'I'm just going to sleep it off'* are all small-scale examples of using an emotional crutch. To put it in basic terms, an emotional crutch is something we have irrationally concluded as something we couldn't live without.

Personally, I don't see too many negatives in enjoying things such as drinking and smoking when in control and when they're a clear, conscious choice. However, when they're solely relied upon as a necessity for everyday life, then you'll find that they are used for reasons that go beyond enjoyment. An emotional crutch is essentially when a 'want' becomes a 'need' - much like an addiction.

A more profound example of an emotional crutch is when anxiety sufferers place so much importance on confining themselves to the walls of their homes. Home is suddenly this overtly safe place, where the walls suddenly become the mechanics of our mind and body's coping mechanisms. It's common to view the outside of the home as this dangerous and overwhelming place that our minds and bodies could not cope with. It's also very common to think that we can deal with our problems within our homes and essentially 'come out when we're ready'.

Emotional crutches are exclusive and subjective to the individual and I suggest that you take time out to distinguish between what you're enjoying and what you're actually relying on. On a personal note, I found that unhealthy habits such as smoking and binge drinking actually made my anxiety feel worse, with it only providing a short term level of enjoyment or escape. Smoking actually over-stimulates the nervous system, making symptoms such as hypersensitivity and panic occur more frequently. Alcohol and the 'hang over' effect also cause similar symptoms and actually place us in states of vulnerability. Drinking alcohol drains our electrolyte levels which puts us at 'risk' of experiencing chest palpitations.

The best way to put yourself to the test with anxiety is to take yourself out of your comfort zone which, in most cases, is our homes. Lose the emotional crutches and see if you can go through a day without them. Of course losing them all at once is a bit much to ask of yourself, so try and cut down on the bad habits a little bit of a time and see how you feel after a week.

If you're feeling agoraphobic, try and spend an hour going for a walk or seeing a friend. Why not cut down the cigarettes or other habitual drugs by half? Cutting down and eventually not having to rely on these emotional crutches did wonders for me when overcoming anxiety.

# Keep Fit, Eat Healthy

Any health professional will tell you that exercise and a healthy diet is paramount when establishing a good bill of health. This applies to dealing with anxiety too. It's well known that exercise and 'feel good' foods help with both physical and psychological ailments. With regards to anxiety, exercise and healthy foods are proven to ease the symptoms it produces. They can help ease symptoms such as heart palpitations, irritable bowel syndrome, poor blood circulation, tiredness and breathlessness to name a few.

Exercise helps to establish a good level of blood circulation, which helps to create efficient oxygen transportation and a good digestive cycle. It also helps the brain to release chemicals such as endorphins, which aid the body to help experience the feeling of being happy and content. It also helps to provide an outlet for excessive adrenaline, which usually comes in abundance for the average anxiety sufferer.

Furthermore, it helps to add structure to our daily lives. Going for a run, cooking a healthy meal, going to the gym, doing household jobs or even going for a walk gives us a daily outlet for any negative feelings and helps to pull us out of negative thought patterns. Doing this, alongside eating healthier foods, has a huge, positive effect on mental health and I seriously recommend it. I believe it would help anyone as much as it greatly helped me.

The old saying of 'you are what you eat' rings true when it comes to choosing the right food. Eating nutritious, healthy foods which contain vitamins, calcium, protein and other essentials, not only aid us physically, but have been proven to help us mentally too. You should take time out to analyse and record which foods have a profound effect on your mood and how they affect you physically.

I decided to drastically cut down on my sugar intake, as well as wheat based products, as I found that they negatively affected my mood and also made me feel bloated. They also made me feel lethargic and unmotivated - leaving me vulnerable for anxious thoughts to creep in. It's different for each individual and must be assessed using your own thoughts and feelings and the observations of those around you.

Here is a list of the common foods that seem to affect those with anxiety:

❖ **Wheat and food with high gluten content. I.e. Bread, dough,** - High wheat and gluten content in foods is known to trigger bloating, the symptoms of Irritable Bowel Syndrome, lethargy, stomach pains and chest tightness.

110

❖ **Sugar in high amounts. I.e. chocolate, sweets, cakes,** - High amounts of sugar intake can be linked to bloating, over-stimulates the nervous system, tiredness, lethargy and headaches.

❖ **Milk products. I.e. butter, cheese, cream,** - Dairy products can affect our digestion, causes I.B.S, bloating, trapped wind, lethargy, headaches and nausea.

❖ **Artificial additives. I.e. 'E numbers', food colourings, sweeteners,** - It takes the body longer to process artificial products. They can cause headaches, nausea, tiredness and can over-stimulate the nervous system.

❖ **Eggs.** - Eggs can drastically affect digestion speed causing indigestion and various other symptoms relating to I.B.S.

❖ **Spices.** - Spicy food can trigger digestion problems and I.B.S.

It's also widely advised that you cut down on red meat, as well as foods containing high fructose. Furthermore, you need to understand that meal sizes, particularly those consisting of large portions, can dramatically affect a person's mood. If we overeat, it causes our bodies to work harder to digest our food - affecting our energy levels.

All of the listed foods have been linked to triggering the symptoms of anxiety and they notably have the ability to lower our overall mood. Wheat and sugar particularly affected my energy levels and digestion, but it's all down to each individual and how their body reacts. For example, you may be affected by dairy products or eggs, but seem fine when eating other foods.

We know that anxiety can cause us to assume the worst case scenario in a given situation. This is important to remember when seeing how our bodies react to foods. During my problems with anxiety, I assumed that I had something far-fetched such as coeliac disease, because I bloated after I ate bread and pizza. Perhaps you get stomach pain after drinking milk, so your anxious brain may assume that you're lactose intolerant.

Just remember that our anxious brains often *need* to find the answer and in doing so will jump to the easiest answer - the worst case scenario. Anxiety has the power to cause I.B.S, bloating, lethargy, stomach pains etc. Just because you have the symptoms of a food intolerance doesn't mean you actually are permanently intolerant. It may just be anxiety. I recommend going to your general practitioner for a food intolerance test for assurance.

Foods which have been shown to provide a positive effect on anxious symptoms and overall mood are:

- ❖ **Fruit** - Bananas, apricots, apples, oranges, tomatoes, blueberries, avocados and various dried fruits such as sultanas, raisins and prunes to name a few.
- ❖ **Vegetables** - Broccoli, spinach, carrots, chickpeas, parsnips, beans, etc.
- ❖ **Nuts and Seeds** - Walnuts, almonds, pistachios, macadamias, Brazil nuts, pumpkin seeds, sunflower seeds, flax seeds, etc.
- ❖ **Grains** - oats, brown rice, corn, barley etc.
- ❖ **Oily fish** - Salmon, tuna, mackerel, sardines, herring etc.

These foods have all been linked to promoting increased mental health. If you're like me and can't resist eating animal meat, then try to stick to lean, white meats such as turkey and perhaps try to eat more fish. Experiment with your diet and record the benefits. This is particularly beneficial when our anxiety levels have improved and we want to continue our development.

# Cut down on caffeine

Caffeine can often be structured into our daily lives and relied upon as a means of providing 'instant' energy. It is a highly addictive stimulant that the body can crave when intake is stopped or lowered. Caffeine can be found in:

- ❖ Coffee
- ❖ Tea
- ❖ Soft Drinks
- ❖ Energy Drinks
- ❖ Painkillers
- ❖ Various medication

For anxiety sufferers, consuming caffeine can be very debilitating, as it can easily trigger off anxious thoughts and symptoms. The aim, particularly with anxiety, is to slowly cut caffeine out of your diet until your anxiety becomes manageable or has subsided. I stress the importance of 'slowly', because those who have a high daily intake of caffeine are at risk of 'caffeine withdrawal'.

Caffeine is a stimulant that increases agitation and anxiety. It's also very acidic, which can lead to inflammation within the body. Caffeine is also a diuretic, which can lead to dehydration and worsen the other symptoms of anxiety.

I often drank coffee and tea as a quick fix to wake up in the morning, or to give myself an afternoon boost to help me focus at work. What I didn't realise was that it actually heightened the feeling of being anxious.

Not only does caffeine provide the feeling of increased energy levels, but it also stimulates our nervous system; this makes us prone to states of hypersensitivity and hyperawareness. We know that these are symptoms of anxiety that we'd much rather avoid. I strongly recommend aiming towards avoiding caffeine altogether and relying on healthier sources of energy such as fruit and high carbohydrate food.

# Patience and discipline

You must be patient when trying to rid yourself of anxiety. If you use patience, perseverance and an alternate life focus, then the anxiety will eventually leave. Do not rush it, but at the same time do not let anxiety define who you are. In order to re-wire your brain to live a better life, you need to establish new habits. This takes time.

This book may have helped you to alleviate your initial fear of anxiety, but in order to truly eradicate it, you need to have a good sense of self-discipline and self-awareness. You need to be able to distinguish between what your true thoughts and beliefs are and that of those that are dictated by anxiety. When we are feeling 'fine', our outlook on life maybe positive and attributes such as our self-esteem, self-belief and motivation may not be questioned. However, when we're feeling anxious, we could think about these same attributes in a more negative light. It is up to you to distinguish which belief that you truly believe in: the positive or the negative.

I think it's very important that you're not too hard on yourself when battling this condition. It's ever too easy to be our own worst critic during anxiety, but you need to realise that you're going through a lot of emotional trauma. There were many times where I thought I was doing well with regards to tackling my anxiety. I'd go weeks abiding by a routine that I knew was healthy for me and that I actually ended up engaging with.

But there were times where I did feel anxious. I did feel the onset of a panic attack. However, I acknowledged that it was simply anxiety trying to creep back in. It did get me down at times and on the odd occasion I felt like crumbling and accepting the label of being an anxious wreck. I persevered though and I insist that you do the same.

So don't whirl up in a panic, or dwell on a depressive state if you feel your anxiety is troubling you. Always focus on the positives and constantly check on how far you've come. I fully believe that everyone with an anxiety disorder can overcome it. You must believe in that too.

# The Do's and Do Not's when approaching anxiety

**Do** - Acknowledge that your symptoms are more than likely connected to an anxiety problem. Group all of your worries under one umbrella and tackle them as one singular problem.

**Do** - Realise that when we feel panicky, lightheaded, wanting to escape or feel like something awful is going to happen, that this is primarily down to adrenaline and other bodily chemicals. The affect of your bodily chemicals have little connection to the outcomes of the outside world. Try and stick it out.

**Do** - Understand that anxiety comes with a lot of symptoms, which at times of high anxiety can seem completely separate from the issue at hand. However, if there is a concern then DO see your general practitioner for reassurance.

**Do -** Partake in what you would usually do or try something new. To begin re-wiring the brain, you must establish new positive thought paths and give the adrenal gland a rest. Do what you would usually do and keep your mind busy!

**Do -** Talk to people and be as open as you can about your anxiety. You'll find that those who care and love you will accept it in their own way and give you the space, time and patience you need to deal with the problem. This is great at relieving any pressures amounting in your social life.

**Do -** Look after your body by keeping it active and providing it with healthy foods.

---

**Do Not -** Accept that anxiety is simply who you are.

**Do Not -** Try to 'think your way out of it' in states of high anxiety. There is no 'miracle thought' that can cure all of your ailments.

**Do Not -** Assume the worst case scenario. Anxiety and panic forces us to do this. Use positive rationalisation to realise that it's probably the anxiety, not your true beliefs.

**Do Not -** Run away from a situation. You'll only place more importance on the issue and make it become a more frightening prospect.

**Do Not -** Rely on emotional crutches, such as the walls of your own home, alcohol, drugs and even smoking.

**Do Not -** Do this alone. Share your thoughts, feelings, progress and experiences with others, regardless of what they think.

**Do Not** - Consume excessive amounts of caffeine and alcohol. Believe me on this one.

# My Story

We have reached this short and somewhat self-indulgent part of the book - my story with anxiety. This part of the book is an optional read, particularly if you're a closet misanthrope like me and cringe at any sign of someone appearing to bask in their own self-involvement. I do feel telling my story is helpful though, as it provides you with an idea about what I went through with my battle with anxiety. It may also provide you with hope as I've been there; I've done it.

My anxiety first started when I left University and was left heavily in debt. I had no job and I was trying to maintain a failing long-distance relationship. I'd also made the decision to quit a pretty destructive cannabis habit (cannabis does not help in the long run).

I felt a bit lost. I didn't know what to do and felt out of my comfort zone. I was worrying about what the future held for me. I was worrying about money, my relationship, where I would live, my old friendships being re-kindled and if I could adapt to my new environment.

It was my first year out of university. I was living with my Mum and younger brother and tried my best to establish myself in the world. I suffered with what can be labeled as *generalised anxiety* and often spent my days dwelling on why I felt so edgy, so different.

I realised that dwelling on my problems wasn't healthy, so I put all of my effort into getting a job, so I could have financial security and an ability to see my partner and my friends more often. It also kept my mind busy.

After a short while, I managed to get a job as a support worker for disabled adults, which I found very rewarding, although there were periods of time in the working day that unfortunately allowed me to dwell on my worries.

After a year, with my worries still the same, I decided that I needed a change. I had almost saved enough money to move into my own place and thought it would help with my generalised anxiety. I loved living with my family, particularly my younger brother, as he was at that fun age of 14 where he helped me to re-live some of my past times, but the mental associations I held about living at home were not helping my anxiety.

I managed to get a better job in a career I always wanted to be involved in. I felt hope. My relationships improved, my anxiety lessened, my social life flourished and I had the opportunity and financial means to move out and start an independent life.

A month before I was due to start my new job, my younger brother was diagnosed with an extremely rare form of cancer. The odds were simply astronomical. My family were in shock and the trauma hit us all hard. I had to stay home and look after my brother and my Mum. The trauma of his diagnosis hit me very, very hard. As for the anxiety, well, I'm sure you can imagine. For 2 years I stayed in my family home and cared for my Mum and brother.

Now I will explain, strictly from an anxiety point of view, what the effects of anxiety did to me during this difficult time. I realise I run the risk of sounding somewhat selfish, given that I wasn't the one with the serious illness, but this book is ultimately about anxiety and I will focus strictly on that.

Immediately after my brother's diagnosis and in my alone time, I began to think and obsess about the concept of death. My main environments were now my home and a children's oncology ward. I was so adamant that I was going to help my brother that I made my whole life about cancer. I wanted to know everything in order to 'save' my brother. Please bare in mind that I already struggled with generalised anxiety.

I couldn't sleep, my brain was in overdrive and all my thoughts about the trauma where on a constant loop. I meticulously analysed and emotionally smothered my brother. I was acting out of panic. Subsequently my relationship with my partner and certain friends broke down. I began to feel more and more isolated, without even acknowledging it, because my focus was so narrow.

After a discussion with my Mum, I decided to proceed to undertake the new job I was due to start, as a means of keeping my mind focused and occupied on other things. This helped my panic-inducing thought patterns ten-fold, but what I failed to do was take some time out to look after myself. My life ultimately ended up being a hectic routine of working, helping my family and dwelling on illness, abandonment and replaying the trauma over and over again in my head. I kept this up for a few months, up until my body had simply had enough.

The breakdown happened.

I was at work one day making myself a hot drink, when all of a sudden I experienced a sudden wave of what can only be described as a complete detachment from my surroundings. My peripheral vision shut down, my breathing altered, my reality appeared distorted and everything seemed more lucid than real. *'What on earth is happening to me?'* I thought.

I began to panic.
It was the start of the mother of all panic attacks.
I was taken home.

For the next five days I locked myself in my room - unable to eat and sleep, experiencing the same level of panic that I had left work with. My mind was in overdrive and I just spent every minute panicking about why I felt the way I did. I couldn't sleep due to excessive worry and often spent my time trying to work out what I was going through. I would not leave the house, speak to anybody or even attempt to do anything that was required in my daily life.

Out of desperation I began to trawl the internet. I attempted to read articles and researched my symptoms everywhere I could find them. Each and every search ended up feeding me a worst case scenario. After two days of feeling perpetually worse, I began to ponder on the possibility that I was going insane - that some incurable, psychological condition was causing my problems and that I was potentially brain damaged. What made it worse was that when I was searching the internet, I had read about many others who were going through the same thing. Some of these people, who had been living with similar symptoms, had been crippled by fear for years.

This added further stress to my already exhausted body. I was trying to fend off the possibility that I was mentally ill, as well as feeling a deep level of guilt about not being able to care for my brother and my Mum. Thoughts just kept playing on loop in my brain. I felt completely immobilised. Then to make things worse, the anxiety started to affect me physically.

I started to get headaches, chest pains, breathing difficulties, heart palpitations, dizziness and this overwhelming sense of being far away from my surroundings. My stomach and ribs began to hurt, I could not keep still and I found focusing on anything to be near impossible. This carried on for weeks. I began to consider giving up. I considered running away (even though I didn't want to leave the house). I considered accepting that I was going insane. I considered suicide and all sorts of thoughts revolving around 'escaping'.

One night, when I was particularly panicky and hadn't slept or ate for three days, I decided to walk to an old friend's house down the road. My friend was surprised when I turned up but allowed me to come in and talk about what I was going through. She listened attentively and after explaining about my predicament, she said something so subtle yet so profound it actually helped to kick start my recovery. *"Well it's no wonder you're having all of this anxiety."* she said.

Of all the racing thoughts and scenario conjurations my mind had processed, not one of them stopped to contemplate that it was just anxiety. Exhausted, I went home and once again tried to piece together a mental puzzle, but I used anxiety as the missing piece. It was a theory that had no flaw. That night I had the best sleep I'd had in a long while.

Don't be under any illusion that all my problems with anxiety suddenly ceased to exist just because I realised that it was 'just anxiety'. What it did do for me was provide me with a platform and a direct and harmless excuse to point all of my problems towards. My life was extremely stressful and I always reminded myself about what my friend said – *'no wonder I'm having all of this anxiety'*. Every time I felt panicky, experienced a physical symptom or noticed that my mind wondered off down a negative thought route, I just blamed it on anxiety.

This was the catalyst for overcoming my excessive anxiety. I did my research, put into practice the strategies and knowhow that you have found in this book and began to just get on with life. I once again became a big help to my family and helped my brother to tackle his illness. I saw friends, my attendance at work significantly improved and I even managed to set some leisure time for myself.

During his illness, I once asked my brother why he never seemed to panic about the severity of the situation. I couldn't understand why I seemed to reach this point of breakdown, whilst he always seemed to keep his cool and get on with things. The truth be told - the boy didn't know. To me he was this immortal figure of endless bravery, with such bravery seemingly a part of him.

After much thought, I realised this belief didn't serve him any justice. The boy actually made the conscious choice to be brave and kept himself mentally healthy through his own actions. This truly inspired me to replicate the same approach. I wanted to be brave and allow my *actions* to dictate my mentality.

I miss him to this day.

There's always hope for this condition. I now live a life almost free from it. I wish you all the best and please feel free to contact me to let me know your own story.

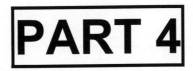

# PART 4

## Emergency Panic Attack Help Page

If you currently feel like you're very anxious, or perhaps are panicking at this very moment, then read on and refer to this page if panic ever strikes again.

OK, so you're panicking...

Let me guess:

Racing thoughts?
Feelings of terror, doom and even fear of death?
Feel like you're going insane?

I know it feels horrible. I've had many panic attacks myself.

You need to realise that **nothing bad is going to happen** to you.

Absolutely nothing.

Your thoughts at this moment in time are merely a projection of your fears.

...this is not the reality of the situation.

You will calm down eventually.

You may not know this but there's a tonne of **adrenaline** and **cortisol** flowing through your veins at this very moment.

They're **harmless bodily chemicals**. You're in no danger.

You have entered **'fight or flight'** mode. You are in no danger.

None at all.

Soon the adrenaline will run out. I know this because the adrenal gland exhausts itself.

Your body can't maintain this panic.

It's biologically impossible.

I'm going to assume that you feel like this panic has come out of nowhere and that it feels out of your control.

You are fine.

**This is normal.**

Do not run away.

It is just the adrenaline. You are in 'fight or flight' mode.

Do you feel very different?

Does everything around you feel different?

They should do, because this is normal at a time like this.

It's just the adrenaline.

Is your mind racing?

A thousand thoughts a second?

Fearing the worst of your predicament?

This is also normal at a time like this.

It's just the adrenaline.

I bet this has happened before, perhaps many a time.

I bet this panic feels just as overwhelming as the other occasions that you've panicked, despite the previous experiences that you've had.

Wherever you are and whatever you're doing, you need to realise that nothing 'bad' is going to happen.

Believe me on this one.

I know how hard it is to 'think straight' when dealing with panic.

All you need to know is that your body has released a lot of harmless adrenaline into your system. Also, your **nervous system** is on **high alert**.

You have entered 'fight or flight' mode.

It's just the adrenaline.

This is normal.

This 'fight or flight' mode causes all sorts of **changes in the mind and body.**

It distorts our reality, makes our **heart beat fast**, makes us **shake, sweat** and **shiver.**

Believe me when I say that adrenaline can cause so many temporary, harmless changes within the body.

It does not matter if you chose to enter fight or flight mode or not. It is happening, and it will pass quickly if you **acknowledge** what is going on within your body.

**Steady your breathing,** let the adrenaline pass and let the **nervous system settle.**

This feeling will pass soon.

Look forward to the fact that when the adrenal gland exhausts itself, it brings a feeling of light euphoria to the mind and body.

Look forward to this - it is a **truly amazing feeling.**

Keep doing what you were supposed to be doing, whether you're at home, at work, travelling or even on holiday.

The feeling will eventually pass.

Do not show this feeling the attention that it does not deserve. Continue with your day and if the feeling ever strikes again, it will not be as intense as this time - I guarantee.

Keep active and **focus on something positive**. This is hard, but even thinking about something positive **diverts the negative thoughts** your mind is homing in on.

Everything will be fine. Nothing bad is going to happen.

Nothing bad *can* happen.

You can do it.

**It's just the adrenaline.**

Printed in Great Britain
by Amazon.co.uk, Ltd.,
Marston Gate.